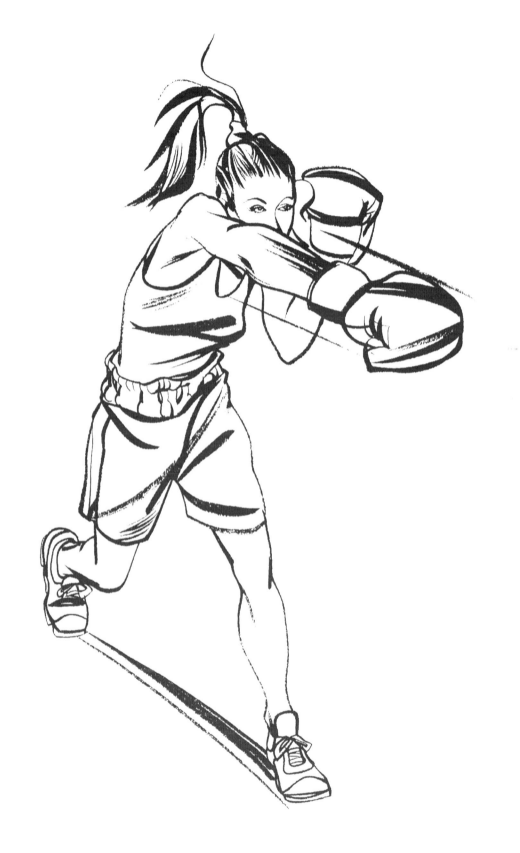

# THE GLEASON'S GYM

## Total Body Boxing Workout for Women

### A 4-Week Head-to-Toe Makeover

**HECTOR ROCA** AND **BRUCE SILVERGLADE**

A FIRESIDE BOOK
Published by Simon & Schuster
New York  London  Toronto  Sydney

FIRESIDE
Rockefeller Center
1230 Avenue of the Americas
New York, NY 10020

This Fireside Edition 2007
FIRESIDE and colophon are registered trademarks
of Simon & Schuster, Inc.

For information regarding special discounts for bulk purchases,
please contact Simon & Schuster Special Sales at 1-800-456-6798
or business@simonandschuster.com.

*Designed by Jaime Putorti*
Interior photographs by Frank Veronsky
Interior illustrations by David Lee / The Studio NYC

Manufactured in the United States of America

10   9   8   7   6   5   4   3   2   1

The Library of Congress has cataloged the hardcover edition as follows:
Roca, Hector.
     The Gleason's Gym : total body boxing workout for women : a 4 week
     head-to-toe makeover / Hector Roca and Bruce Silverglade
          p.    cm.
     1. Boxing—Training.  2. Physical fitness.  I. Silverglade, Bruce.  II. Title.
     GV1137.6.R63    2006
     796.83—dc22                          2006048308

ISBN-13: 978-0-7432-8687-9
ISBN-10:      0-7432-8687-1
ISBN-13: 978-0-7432-8688-6 (Pbk)
ISBN-10:      0-7432-8688-X (Pbk)

★ I want to dedicate this workout book to Gleason's Gym and its wonderful tradition and history.

*Hector Roca*

★ I want to dedicate this workout book to the great guys that made Gleason's Gym what it is today: Bobby Gleason and Ira Becker.
And of course to my wonderful and loving wife, JoEllen VanOuwerkerk, who is my real inspiration.

*Bruce Silverglade*

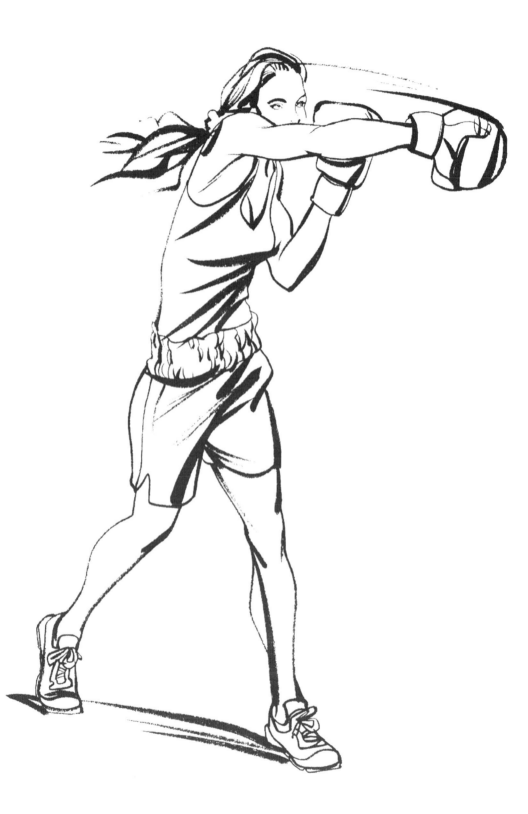

# Contents

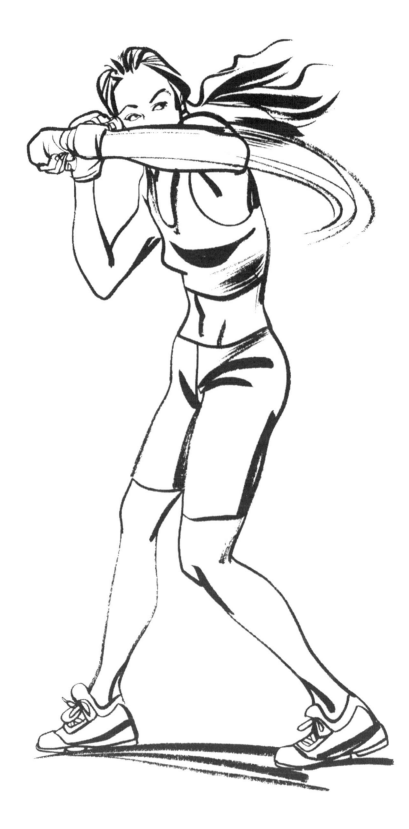

# Foreword

I remember getting on the subway at the corner of Eighth Avenue and Fourteenth Street and getting off at High Street in Brooklyn on my way to Gleason's. The ride over was always filled with excitement over what my day at the gym would bring. What obstacle would I face? What challenge would Hector present me with? What would my mind and body have to overcome?

Walking through the doors of the gym brought a rush of adrenaline that I knew would carry me through whatever would be thrown at me—literally.

At Gleason's, I worked, cried, laughed, fell, got up, sweated, lost bad weight, gained good weight, got punched, punched back. And every day when I walked out of those doors and got back on the subway, I knew a little bit more about myself and what I was capable of. It was more than I ever knew to dream.

I wish the same for you.

*—Hilary Swank*

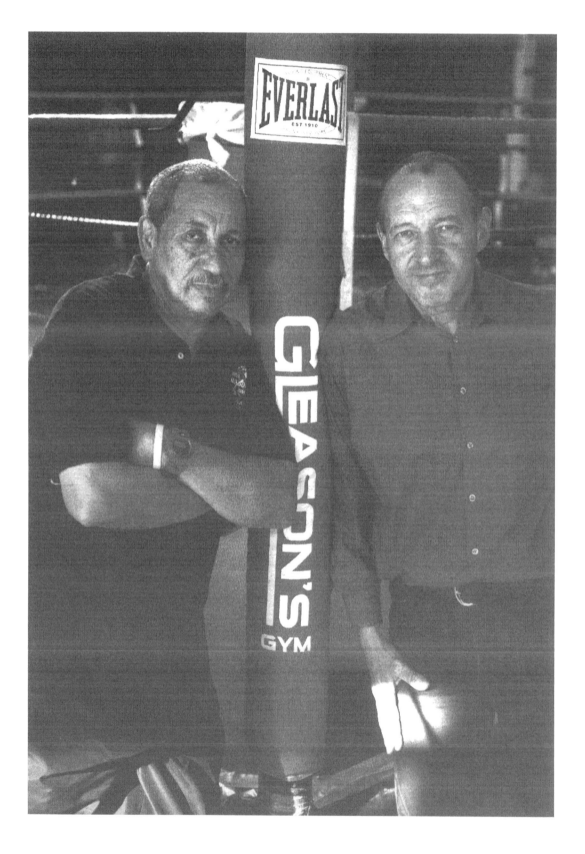

# Introduction

THE HISTORY OF GLEASON'S GYM

**Bruce Silverglade, owner**

In the South Bronx, during the Great Depression, boxing was known as an Irishman's sport, which is why a little-known Italian bantamweight named Peter Robert Gagliardi changed his name to Bobby Gleason before opening the doors of his boxing gym in 1937.

For $50 a month, Gleason, forty-five, rented a decrepit but sunny second-floor loft in an old factory building on the corner of 149th Street and Westchester Avenue. Looking out its eight-foot windows, the fighters could see the Royal Theater, where vaudeville stars, including Sophie Tucker, performed; the Central Theater, where neighborhood kids could buy a candy bar and catch a triple feature for a dime; and the Bronx Opera House, the neighborhood's grand dame.

Dues at the gym were $2 a month, and Gleason put up a tough front when it came to collecting them. He hung a sign in his office that read, "Your dues are due today. If they have not been paid, please do so and save yourself the embarrassment of being asked." Despite the notice, he let many of his struggling fighters slide for months. Barely able to afford the gym himself, Gleason hacked a cab for ten to twelve hours a night, seven days a week.

With his savings, Gleason outfitted the place with four heavy bags, six racks to hang speed bags (fighters had to bring their own), and a full-sized ring surrounded by chairs for spectators. The locker rooms consisted of one toilet and two showers, which only worked in the winter. (In the summer, the neighborhood kids would cool off by running through the water that came from the city fire hydrants, which sapped the gym's water pressure.) Summer, you can imagine, was not easy on the nose.

Despite its quirks, Gleason's quickly became home to a deep roster of world champions, including Jake "Raging Bull" LaMotta; Mike Belloise; Phil Terranova, who Gleason managed; and Jimmy Carter. Thanks to their charisma, boxing's popularity surged, and Gleason's reputation for turning out top contenders grew. Six days a week, morning until night, the great trainers of the day—Patty Colovito, Freddie Brown, Chickie Ferrara, and Charlie Galeta—plied their craft inside—and the crowds followed. There was *never* a still punching bag or free space left on the floor for shadowboxing or skipping rope. The wait to get into the ring, which was first-come, first-serve, often topped out at nearly two hours.

Throughout the forties and fifties, Gleason's, as well as two of the city's other boxing institutions, Stillman's and the Old Garden, flourished, but by the sixties, "Boxing's Golden Age" had ended. With no attention-grabbing boxers, the sport's popularity receded. Bobby Gleason managed to hang onto his gym, while Stillman's and the Old Garden went down for the count.

Gleason's remained the permanent training base for many world champs, and many out-of-town contenders, including Walter Cartier and Joe Frazier, set up their temporary base in the Bronx when they had fights scheduled at Madison Square Garden. In 1964, Muhammad Ali, then known as Cassius Clay, trained at Gleason's for his fight with Sonny Liston. (That fight was one of the biggest upsets of the twentieth century; Ali won the World Heavyweight title when Liston failed to answer the bell in the seventh round.) Later, Panamanian superman Roberto

Duran used Gleason's to win three world titles. When Duran was at the gym, so seemingly was the rest of New York. Oftentimes, the surrounding street would have to be blocked off to accommodate all of his fans.

In 1974, after thirty-seven years on Westchester Avenue, Bobby Gleason, then eighty-two, put a lock on the Bronx gym door for good. The building was knocked down, and a housing project was constructed in its place. Gleason moved his establishment to Thirtieth Street and Eighth Avenue in Manhattan, and renowned trainers Ray Arcel, Freddy Brown, and Whitey Bimstein followed him to the new location. It was the first street-level gym in New York City. It came well-equipped with an L-shaped mezzanine for the crowds, two training rings, six heavy bags, separate rooms for shadowboxing and skipping rope, and even a luncheonette.

Seven years later, in his late eighties, Bobby Gleason passed away, and Ira Becker, a long-time boxing supporter and staunch safety regulator, took over. Membership tripled, and the gym's great tradition continued on. World champions, including Hector Camacho, Julio Cesar Chavez, Riddick Bowe, Larry Holmes, Michael Spinks, Mike Tyson, and "Gentleman Gerry" Cooney, trained at the Manhattan location.

Hollywood scriptwriters followed. Martin Scorcese and Robert Deniro shot *Raging Bull* at the gym. Other movies filmed on site include *Midnight Run, The Ten Count, Heart,* and *Rage of Angels.*

In early 1983, I struck a deal with Ira Becker to become his partner and half-owner of Gleason's on a part-time basis. Boxing runs in my family. My father was a cofounder of the National PAL, and he later managed the 1980 and 1984 U.S. Olympic boxing teams. After a tough divorce I'd thrown myself into the sport in 1976 and began refereeing and judging amateur bouts. I'd caught the boxing bug, and soon I quit my sixteen-year post at Sears Roebuck and Company to run Gleason's full-time.

In 1984, the Thirtieth Street building turned co-op, and Gleason's was forced to move to its current location, a converted warehouse off a cobblestone street under the Brooklyn Bridge. While the surroundings and equipment have changed since 1937 (the 15,000-square-foot gym now has ten heavy bags and four full-sized rings), the fighting spirit remains. To date, 126 world champions have called Gleason's home, including Arturo Gatti, Junior Jones, Buddy McGirt, Kevin Kelly, Alicia Ashley, and sizzling welterweight Zab Judah. World-class contenders David Telesco, Oleg Maskaev, Yuri Foreman, Raul Frank, Wayne Braithwaite, and Vivian Harris currently train at the gym. Gleason's is also proud of its amateur champions: In the first National Amateur Women's tournament, Gleason's sent six contestants, and they each returned with a gold medal.

Over the past seven decades, Gleason's gym has become synonymous with excellence in boxing. And for the first time in history, boxing has reached the masses, as investment bankers, fashion models, and actors join the gym to train alongside professional fighters.

Wesley Snipes, Jennifer Lopez, Michelle Rodriguez, John Leguizamo, and Harry Connick Jr. have all stepped into our ring. Most recently, Hilary Swank trained here with boxing's elderstatesman Hector Roca for her role in *Million Dollar Baby*.

Boxing is a sport of the underdog, and people have used it to fight their way out of hopelessness. When you spend a little time in Gleason's, even as a spectator, you feel this. There's a true sense of equality and acceptance because all the members identify themselves as fighters, first and foremost. After that, all their other differences fade into the background. That's incredible, considering that our membership represents sixty-seven different nationalities.

The welcoming atmosphere is one of the things I love most about Gleason's. In a lot of ways, Gleason's is a microcosm of society: a gritty melting pot characterized by openness and acceptance and inhabited by a lot of people with big dreams. Whether you're working out or just watching, a professional or an amateur, you are respected in this house.

There is a quote by Virgil painted in black on the red walls of our gym: "Now whoever has courage, and a strong and collected spirit in his breast, let him come forward, lace on the gloves and put up his hands." These words resonate throughout the gym, and they are what Gleason's still stands for today.

# THE GLEASON'S GYM

## Total Body Boxing

## Workout for Women

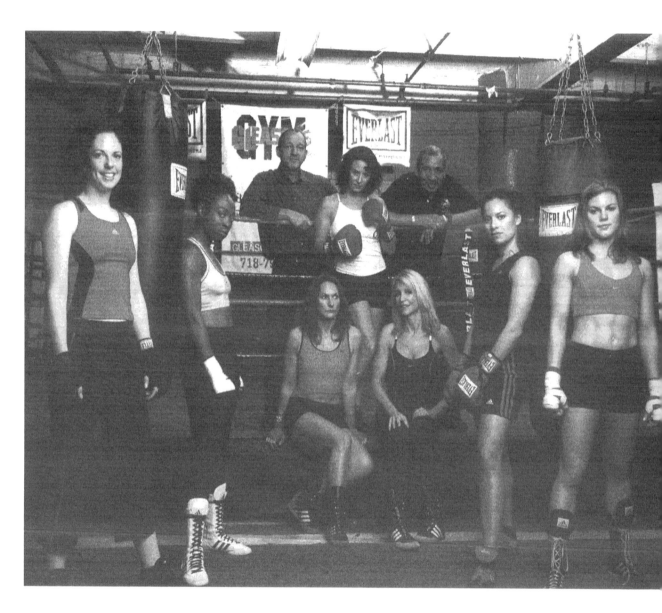

# 1

# Gleason's
# Total Body Makeover:
## About the Program

**A**lthough Gleason's Gym has been around for years, boxing has gone mainstream, particularly among women for the first time ever. Thanks in large part to the success of the movie *Million Dollar Baby,* boxing has made a knockout entrance into today's zeitgeist. Even if Hilary Swank's *Million Dollar Baby* acceptance speech fades in the audience's memory, the sight of her *Million Dollar* abs and biceps never will. Just as yoga burst into popularity in the 1990s and Pilates caught on the early 2000s, boxing is now taking center ring.

But beyond the Hollywood spotlight, there's something deeper behind the sport's popularity. In a world where there's so much hype, so many half-truths, and so many fake fixes for real problems, boxing acts as an emotional and physical leveler, where only the truly toughest, fastest, fittest, and strongest make it. This frankness of the sport makes it so refreshing and appealing. Work hard, and you *will* succeed. Fake it, and you won't. "I see so many parallels between boxing and life," Swank told *Sports Illustrated.* "You have to stay in the moment, or you get hit. You have to let everything go. . . . and you have to stay humble."

Now, here's the good news: You don't have to live in Brooklyn or have a movie-star salary to train with Hollywood's number one boxing trainer. Hector Roca, who's coached thirteen world champions, has put together this four-week, one-on-one training program loosely based on Swank's muscle-molding regimen.

While Swank trained for nearly thirty hours a week, you'll train for thirty to forty-five minutes a day for four weeks to achieve your total body makeover. And while that may not be enough to get you ready for the Golden Gloves (or the Golden Globes), it's certainly enough to make you look and feel like a winner. In fact, after working out for up to forty-five minutes, three days a week, for four weeks, you'll reap the total body makeover rewards, which include:

## • You'll get lean and lose weight.

It's a simple matter of math. You will burn more calories in a shorter period of time than you ever have before. Your waist will become smaller, and your clothes will become looser.

"I lost 20 pounds, and now I have a focus and a goal."
—Jill Emery, age 35

## • You'll boost your cardiovascular fitness.

Everyday tasks, such as carrying your groceries or running up stairs, will suddenly feel easier because your heart will be stronger and your lung capacity will increase. You'll have more energy than ever before. And you'll be quicker, snappier, and more agile.

"Every three-minute round of boxing is like an hour of aerobics."
—Amy Bridges, age 49, who drives into Brooklyn every day from Greenwich, Connecticut, to train at Gleason's.

# You'll build strength and define your muscles.

Boxing is a total body workout. First you'll see improved definition in your biceps, triceps, and shoulders. Many of the women who train with us are happy to see these results quickly, and they start wearing tank tops that show off their sleek shoulders. You'll uncover your inner six-pack abs, and your legs, from the constant motion, will lean down and firm up. And all of this will be happening simultaneously. Bottom line: You'll see big changes in your body as you begin to train.

"When I first started boxing, I was unable to lift 3-pound weights above my head for more than a few times. Now I have lost weight, am much better toned, and have a lot more confidence. And I can pick up my 54-pound pit bull with ease!"

—Leila Ferioli, age 43

# You'll improve your overall health.

The resistance training in boxing—the push-ups, the squats, and other core strength exercises—strengthen your bones and help prevent osteoporosis. The cardiovascular drills help lower cholesterol and fight fatigue. Regular exercisers sleep better, and all our boxers at Gleason's become good sleepers.

"Since I started boxing, I've become more health-conscious, much more aware of what I put in my body. As a nurse, I'm on my feet all day, dealing with patients and their families, and getting in the ring after work is a great way to unwind. I've found muscles I never knew I had. I can lift and transfer patients much more easily now."

—Jean Marie Reisman, RN, age 25

# You'll feel less stressed.

Not only will boxing help release tension and anxiety—there's nothing more cathartic than visualizing punching your boss in the nose—but it'll also give you a new sense of self-confidence and accomplishment. Unlike no-pain, no-gain fitness routines, boxing is just plain fun.

"I fell in love with boxing four years ago when I came to Gleason's to watch a friend. Now when I'm boxing, my day goes better. I drain myself of any stress or negative energy that the world puts on me."

—Alexis Asher, age 23

## • You'll feel safer.

Many moves you will learn in this book are the same moves you'd learn in a self-defense class. You will be faster, stronger, and know how and where to punch someone if need be.

"I am stronger mentally and spiritually, and I have a much stronger sense of myself. Boxing has made me ready for any challenge, in or out of the ring. No one can break me unless I allow them to."

—Ann-Marie Saccurato, age 28

To do this workout, you do *not* have to be a boxer. You do not have to hit anybody or be hit. You do not have to join an expensive gym. You do not have to buy any expensive equipment. You only need a jump rope. In fact, you don't even have to leave your living room. *The Gleason's Gym Total Body Workout for Women* will lay out a step-by-step, four-week training program that you can do, regardless of your current fitness level. Boxing is 50 percent mental, 40 percent conditioning, and 10 percent skill combined with 100 percent dedication. All you need to begin with is the dedication. We'll take care of everything else, and in four weeks (and four chapters), we'll have you in knockout shape—fitter, faster, and firmer than ever.

It all begins with mental fitness. This is your chance to train with the best, the gym that has trained 126 world champions, and many, many more world-class contenders and amateur champs. We will teach you how to commit, to focus, and to dedicate yourself to the sport and to your body. Next you will learn how to build a strength and aerobic-fitness base and how to eat right and take care of your body as you prepare to box. Then we'll share Hector's basics of boxing—how to stand, punch, and defend yourself.

In the four workout chapters, Hector lays out each week's workouts that make up this four-week program. You will practice the very same moves that Roca's fighters practice in Gleason's Gym every day. If you want to take your skills to the next level and get into ring-ready shape, there will be a plan to help you advance your skill, in which Roca will give advice on how to continue your boxing workout.

Learning to box through the method taught at America's oldest boxing gym is a unique opportunity. Gleason's is a sweat and hard-work gym, old-school with few frills. We've built our success on the experience, knowledge, and skills of our trainers, most notably, Hector Roca. Although you may never set foot into a boxing ring or even a boxing gym, at the end of our workout, you will have the strength, stamina, and skills to really fight. That's what we are offering; the rest is up to you. What you bring to the table are desire and determination. So be serious, pay attention, work hard, stick to it, and stay focused. Time after time, we've seen that's what it takes to be a champion.

Turn the page and get started.

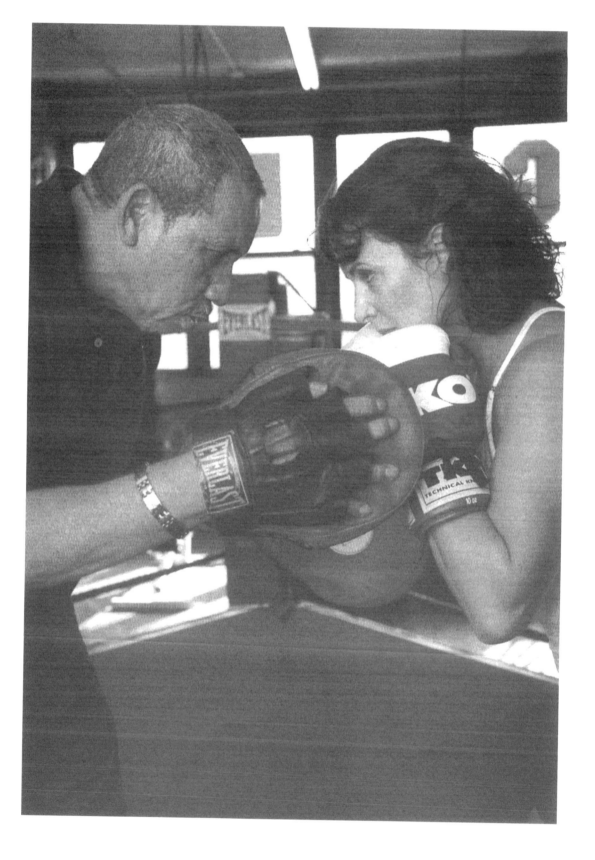

# 2
# Mental Preparation:
## Are You Ready?

The difference between *saying* you're a fighter and actually *being* a fighter is mostly in your head. Mental commitment is the key to all of your life goals. So whether you reach your goals or just fall short, whether you achieve (and keep) your target weight or struggle and yo-yo back and forth, whether you live up to your potential or just get by all depends on your dedication to your own success, your courage to take risks, and your determination to follow through. You can call yourself a fighter, but you can't be one if you don't plan on doing the work.

When it comes to boxing, half of the fight takes place in your mind. The sport is 50 percent mental, 40 percent conditioning, and only 10 percent skill—and *anybody* can learn the skill. At Gleason's, we've made fighters of men and women of *all* shapes, sizes, and backgrounds. Our youngest fighter is seven. Our oldest is seventy-eight. They box because they have the desire to live a better life—to be fitter, stronger, sexier, and less-stressed. Everybody has their own reason to box, and you must find yours before you start.

Boxing is like a marriage. You don't get married just because everybody else has. You have to *like* your spouse. You don't box because everyone else does. You have to *like* it. That's the only way you can do it. If you like it, it's easy.

## ★ WHY DO YOU BOX? ★

*Some women of Gleason's Gym
explain why they love the sport.*

"Boxing, at the beginning, was just a way to get in shape, learn something new and have fun. But then I saw other women competing, and I thought, 'I can do that!' It has made me so competitive that I want to win the Golden Gloves. I've only competed once and I lost in the semifinals, but next year I plan to get the Gold. I want to tell my children that when you work hard at something, this is what you get."

—Angela, age 31

"I box to learn discipline, focus, and skill, and I do it for the romance. Boxing is such a huge part of the American culture, and I want to be a part of a storied tradition."

—Emily, age 31

"I box because I love the science of the sport. And I think it's the ultimate sport, because there are no balls or goals or props. It's just two people using their brains, hearts, and bodies."

—Golden Gloves winner Geneve Brossard, age 28

> "I box because it's a passion and dream of mine to reach the highest limits."
> —Maureen Shea, 24, Hilary Swank's sparring partner during her training for Million Dollar Baby

> "I box because it makes me feel powerful and in control of my life. I can release a lot of anger and frustrations from my body and channel my energy in a positive direction."
> —Lawson, age 39

# Test Your Motivation:
# Five Questions to Ask Yourself Before You Begin

## 1. How badly do you want results?

Muhammad Ali, who trained for his 1965 fight against Sonny Liston at Gleason's, said it best: "Champions aren't made in gyms. Champions are made from something they have deep inside them—a desire, a dream, a vision. They have to have last-minute stamina, they have to be a little faster. They have to have the skill and the will, but the will must be stronger than the skill." If you want to change your body, you can't just give it lip service. You must have the desire to be a champion. You have to want to lose the weight. You have to want to tone your muscles. You have to be willing to do whatever it takes to achieve your goals.

## 2. Do you have the courage to take risks?

Ali also said, "He who is not courageous enough to take risks will accomplish nothing in life." Making a change is scary because it means you're opening yourself up to the possibility of success or failure. Accept that you *will* make mistakes during your journey to becoming a boxer. Everyone does. The difference between a true fighter and a faker is that a fighter views her mistakes as learning experiences, as challenges to becoming better. The faker sees mistakes as failures and gives up. Don't give up. Have confidence in yourself. And remember, you have the Gleason's fighters supporting you.

## 3. Are you dedicated to making changes?

This is a short program. It's hard, but it's not too hard. It requires some time, but it doesn't require a lot of time. It is tough but it doesn't require deprivation. What it does require is a commitment from you to *follow through*. You have to want to learn to be a fighter and be committed to practicing and working hard. If you just go through the motions for thirty or forty-five minutes a day, three days a week, you're not going to get anywhere. If you're dedicated to learning the skills and putting in the effort every day, to live better and push yourself a little harder, maybe harder than you've ever pushed yourself, you're going to see results.

## 4. Do you trust your trainer?

When boxers step into the ring, they're standing twenty-four inches away from someone who is trying to harm them. The last seconds of a match are just as challenging as the first seconds of a match, so there is no "winding down." You have to learn to go the distance. Boxers put their lives on the line through their trainer's instructions, and they have to believe in him enough to say to themselves, "If I do what he tells me, I won't get hurt—and I'll win." Even if you have no intention of actually sparring, you still have to trust your trainer. If you do what we say, you're not going to get hurt, and you will grow into a real fighter.

## 5. Are you ready to step into the ring and willing to take punches?

Fighting is not a one-way street. You must be willing to defend yourself, to take a punch, and to give one. In fact, getting hit should precipitate your counterpunch. You should develop a rhythm of give and take. Therefore, you do not have time to overthink the event. You will never be fast enough if you do. Thinking about it comes after when you are analyzing the fight; hopefully your victory.

# ★ CHOOSE YOUR FIGHT SONG! ★

*Music is a great motivator. It helps you work harder and longer. Here are some of our favorite songs to listen to while boxing.*

1. *Fight the Power,* Public Enemy

2. *Mama Said Knock You Out,* LL Cool J

3. *Get Your Freak On,* Missy Elliot

4. *I Love Rock 'n' Roll,* Joan Jett and the Blackhearts

5. *Kid's Allright,* Bettie SerVeert

6. *Been Caught Stealing,* Jane's Addiction

7. *Deceptacon,* Le Tigre

8. *Rough,* Queen Latifah

9. *Do Your Best,* Femi Kuti, featuring Mos Def

10. *Funkier Than a Mosquito's Tweeter,* Nina Simone

11. *Apparently Nothin',* Young Disciples

12. *Ray of Light,* Madonna

13. *Fighter,* Christina Aguilera

14. *A Stroke of Genuis,* Freelance Hellraiser

15. *Love Spreads,* The Stone Roses

16. *Mrs. Leroy Brown,* Loretta Lynn

17. *Tough Mary,* Etta James

18. *Hit Me With Your Best Shot,* Pat Benetar

19. *Eye of the Tiger,* Survivor

## Visualize Success

If you watch boxing on TV, often it just looks like two people, standing two feet apart, pummeling each other. Sometimes, unfortunately, that's all it is, but better fighters treat the match like a dance, with each opponent struggling to lead. You have to be sharp enough to make your opponent go where you want him or her to go. You should always know your next move and five moves ahead of that. Big time boxers see psychologists before high-stakes bouts. They visualize the entire fight before they step into the ring. They know exactly what they're going to do throughout the fight, so they can make their opponents do what they want them to do.

Visualization is an excellent tool for you, too. You may not step into the ring anytime soon (or ever), but to help you succeed, you should focus on what you want to do. Think about how you want your body to move. Visualize your heart pumping blood to feed your muscles. See yourself throwing rapid-fire punch combinations. Feel your abs contract with each jab. Feel light on your feet. Picture how you're going to look in four weeks. If ever you feel tired or weak or your head isn't in it, visualize your success. It is well within your reach. All you have to do is *want it.*

## Shut the Door on Your Demons

The biggest obstacle to getting fit is not lack of time, or money, or anything else you can think up. Those are just excuses. What keeps people from investing in their own bodies is a lack of self-worth. Get this straight right now: You deserve to be healthy. You deserve to be happy. You deserve a fair shot to work for the life that you want. It takes hard work. Boxing isn't easy. Especially if you're not sparring, and it's just you and your mirror—you're working against yourself. Deep down inside you have to want to find success and know that you deserve it.

Demons plague every boxer. If anyone tells you otherwise, they're lying. Fighters get extremely emotional before their fights because they're actually entering combat. The demons slip into your mind about an hour before the fight, while you're sitting alone in your dressing room, thinking about the match. You start to wonder if the other fighter has trained harder than you. You think about that day you just coasted through your workout, knowing your opponent went all out. You remember the morning you ran four and a half miles when your trainer told you to run five. You remember that night you polished off a pizza when you were supposed to be eating lean. Fighting those demons is what makes boxing a mental, as well as physical, sport.

Maybe you're not preparing for a match. What if you're boxing to get in shape for a big day—your wedding, your class reunion, a big presentation at work? The demons will come for you, too. As you're putting on your clothes, you start to wonder what you'd look like if you did the full ten minutes of cardio, rather than stopping at eight minutes. Or if you had really focused on your form while shadowboxing, instead of just half-heartedly going through the motions. You remember spooning that entire pint of Ben & Jerry's in front of the television and wonder how much better you'd feel right now if you'd kept it in moderation. These are your demons. This is your mental battle.

The difference between a world champion and every other boxer is the same difference between a person who feels 100 percent proud of their body and someone who feels embarrassed in a bathing suit. The winners can stop their own demons before they even enter. Their secret is very simple: Listen to your trainers. Do what we say. If we told you to run for ten minutes straight and you did it, you're ready for the challenge. If you cheated, then you haven't fulfilled your full potential, and you'll always wonder if you've done enough or how much better you could do.

Follow the program. Don't slack. If you do everything we ask you to do, you will reach your goal. And remember, it's only four weeks. It's not hard. There's no guesswork. You can do it. Don't let your demons tell you otherwise.

## — COACH'S CORNER —

Be hungry! Be somebody!

I once had a young fighter who kept saying, "I'm going to lose; I'm going to lose." I used reverse psychology and said, "I want you to lose. Just have fun." This relieved her from the stress of competition, and she went into the ring not caring about winning—and won her bout.

I don't expect my fighters to give up. I say, "Why did you start?" When you start something, you must finish. There is no other choice.

# Control Your Fear

We once had an ultramarathoner train at Gleason's. She could run 100 miles straight without even feeling tired. She was in top physical condition, which is why she wanted to go into the ring to spar right away. After one three-minute round, she was doubled over, panting. Why? She wasn't in top *mental* condition. She could jog forever and feel clear-headed and happy, but when we put someone in front of her who wanted to punch her, her fear started flowing and exhausted her.

Fear is the biggest energy zapper in the ring, and the only way to overcome it is to have faith in your trainer and in yourself. The only way to know if you're demon-proof and if you're strong enough to overcome your fears is to look in the mirror. You're the only person in the world who really knows what you've done and whether you gave it all you had. You cannot lie to yourself.

Sometimes the best way to get rid of fear is to control it. Your opponent is afraid also. Everyone has fear. It is better to confront it and turn it into an outward display of anxious aggression than to submerge it and let it eat at you and undermine your fight plan. Be intelligent.

## — FIGHTING WORDS —

"To be a great champion you must believe you are the best. If you're not, pretend you are."—Muhammad Ali

# ★ FEND OFF FATIGUE ★

*Here are a few other energy-boosting tricks*
*to try when you're feeling beat.*

1. Chew peppermint gum. Maybe you've heard about how Olympic weightlifters take a whiff of smelling salts before hoisting a heavy load. The same principle holds true with peppermint gum, but it's a lot more enjoyable. Pop a piece of peppermint gum before your workout, and you'll fend off fatigue. The scent stimulates the irritant nerve, which helps induce wakefulness, and therefore, allows you to work harder. Of course, spit it out before you step into the ring.

2. Eat strawberries. Research shows the smell of berries helps you burn more calories during your workout (buttered popcorn, too, strangely enough).

3. Ritualize relaxation. Negative thoughts drain your energy faster than anything else. If you tell yourself you can't do something, you won't succeed. It's that simple. So to eliminate those nagging thoughts from your mind before you start working out, try this relaxation ritual: Close your eyes and take ten deep breaths, inhaling and exhaling to your lungs' full capacity. Picture positive, strong energy entering your body as you breath, in and imagine weakness, fatigue, and negative thoughts leaving your body as you exhale.

4. Regroup and restart. We all have those days when just thinking about working out, let alone actually doing it, feels totally exhausting. It's ok to have those days. After all, we all have lives that can get in the way of our workouts. Still, it's important to ask yourself, "Why do I feel this way?" and address the problem. If you're sick, go get some rest. If you're emotionally tired from a fight you just had with your partner, go make up. You're not going to be able to focus your energy on your training if your mind is elsewhere. Once you address the problem, you'll be able to dedicate yourself more fully to your workout.

"A champion shows who he is by what he does when he's tested. When a person gets up and says 'I can still do it,' he's a champion." —Evander Holyfield

# Set Goals

It's probably safe to assume that you picked up this book because you want something more out of your life. Maybe you want to be a world champion boxer. Maybe you want to lose a few pounds. Maybe you want to get stronger. Maybe you want to become active. Whatever your motive, it's important to be clear, specific, and realistic about your ambitions. Exercising without goals is like getting in your car and driving without any idea of where you're going. Without a destination, how do you know you're even headed in the right direction?

Goals set your mind in motion so your body can follow. When you're tired, sweaty, and sore, you're going to ask why you're putting yourself through this. If you don't have an immediate answer to that question, you're going to quit. What's more, only specific types of goals provide enough incentive to actually keep exercisers inspired for the long haul. Here are some tips for setting goals fit for champions.

Be specific. When you're eking out your eighth push-up and your arms are shaking and sweat is rolling off your nose and you want nothing more than to be sitting on your couch watching *Desperate Housewives*, which thought would more likely keep you going: I want to help protect myself against heart disease, or I told myself I'd do ten push-ups today and I'm going to do them? Explicit goals work better than general ones at keeping you motivated.

Be reasonable. If you've never boxed before, then it's highly unlikely that by the time you get to chapter 10, you'll be ready to beat Zab Judah or Maureen Shea, Hilary Swank's sparring partner. Setting impossible goals is just as unproductive as not setting goals at all. Give yourself a reality check and then set yourself up for success by setting goals that are actually attainable. And don't be afraid to take baby steps. Starting any new routine too hard can lead to burn out.

Be nearsighted. Focus your goals on the here-and-now rather than the outcome. Think in terms of jumping rope for five more minutes a week, rather than say, losing ten pounds in one month. You'll feel more satisfied every time you achieve a day-to-day objective, even if it's small, and the happier you feel, the more likely you'll be to stick with it.

Be focused. Exercise certainly benefits your life in more ways than one, and it's important to remind yourself of that in order to stave off boredom. Each day, in addition to setting your progress goals, make it a point to focus on how each move is helping you. Think, I'm boxing to strengthen my bones. I'm boxing to lose weight. I'm boxing to help my heart. I'm boxing to boost my mood. I'm boxing to release my anger. You can go through this entire program without repeating the same motivation.

Be self-observant. Get a notebook and write down your goals and how you felt after you achieved each one. When your motivation is flagging, you can read your exercise journal and remember why you're working so hard.

Be imaginative. Sometimes, just for the heck, of it imagine you are Muhammad Ali, dancing and jabbing. Imitate his style. Adopt his psyche or take the opposite—imitate Joe Frazier. Get low, hook. Be whomever you want—let your imagination fly.

# Make Exercise a Habit

It's difficult to start any new exercise program, especially if your body isn't used to moving every day. But if you take certain steps, you can actually train your body to crave exercise. You will like working out, instead of dreading it. Here's what to do to get in gear.

1. **Make a date with yourself.** In fact, make three this week right now. Get out your calendar and—in pen—put three thirty-minute chunks of time on hold for you to do Week One's workouts. It helps if you block out consistent times, say, every day at 6:00 P.M. You'll get used to clearing your schedule, and soon exercising at that time will become a no-brainer.

2. **Get out your wallet.** Money is a great motivator. Spending a little dough on something actually gives you incentive to follow through. So, don't be afraid to splurge on a new workout outfit, new sneakers, and/or some boxing gloves. If it helps you feel the part, it can help exercise feel like a part of you.

3. **Focus on the positive.** Nobody is making you exercise. You choose to do it. Tell yourself that before you workout. Then concentrate on all the parts of your workout that make you feel great. Think about how strong your shoulders feel when you deliver a right cross. Think about how you love the challenge of jumping rope. Think about how happy it makes you to see that little ridge on the back of your upper arm, aka your tricep, pop out for the first time.

4. **Always cool down.** If you take five to ten minutes to cool down after your workout, you'll be likely to stick with the program. Research shows that people who do post-workout cool downs associate more positive feelings with their exercise programs, both immediately afterward and also in the long run, than those who do not. Of course, the happier you feel about your workout, the less likely you'll be to skip it.

5. **Pay attention to your body, not your weight.** If you're feeling proud of your footwork, your jabs, your dedication, do *not* check your progress by the numbers—at least not yet. That means, for the first four weeks of the workout, no scale. No body fat calipers. No trying on your skinny jeans. Here's why: Research shows that women, in particular, tend to feel better about their bodies and have a higher self-image sooner than the numbers indicate. Translation: You'll probably feel like you've lost weight before you actually have. That's not a bad thing. In fact, those good feelings will keep you motivated throughout the entire workout. When you complete it, just four weeks from now, *then* go ahead and take all the measurements you want. You'll be pleased with the results.

6. **Create a support network.** The boxers at Gleason's turn to one another every day for support. It's important to build your own circle of friends and family who will root you on, as you become a boxer. Be sure that your friends, family, and spouse are behind you in your goal to get in shape and to do it by boxing. Explain to them why you're doing this and why it's important to you. Make them understand that you are committed and driven. There will be people in your life who will think you're crazy for wanting to be a fighter. Don't listen to them. Turn instead to people who believe in you and what you're doing.

7. **Recognize the negative.** Think of the worse that can happen to you—you can lose or get hurt. We have all lost before and, as for getting hurt, boxing injuries during training are not incapacitating. In the past twenty-six years at Gleason's Gym, there has never been a serious injury. The EMS has responded to only a case of dehydration and a sprained ankle.

# ★ SECRET SOURCES OF MOTIVATION ★

Our fighters are motivated by success. Winners want to win again. And once you start training and you notice how good you look and feel, how strong you've become, and how much stamina you have, you'll want to push yourself and train harder so that you can move to your own next level.

But some days you may just feel tired, or you may feel like you can't throw one more punch, do one more sit up, or jump rope for another minute. Here's how some of our fighters dig deep.

"I follow a training schedule no matter how tired I am. Once I start moving, I work through feeling tired. It's always worth it. I had breast cancer five years ago, but I never stopped training, even after my surgery and during radiation. It felt great, and I credit my fast recovery to being in such good shape."                                   —JoEllen VanOuwerkerk, age 48

"I just think about how hard my opponent is training, which makes me train ten times as hard."                                   —Maureen Shea, age 24

"I just convince myself that if I don't even try to [work out], even if it's just for a short time, I will feel grumpy, lazy, and mad at myself. That's how I push myself to get to the gym when I don't want to."       —Angela, age 31

"I have fantasies about glory in the ring, and I turn my sweat and pain into devotion."                                   —Emily, age 31

"I listen to the sounds of the gym and then play the Chemical Brothers on my iPod when I start skipping rope. In about one minute, all my tiredness just disappears."                                   —Lawson, age 39

# Believe

All good boxers believe in something, whether it's themselves, God, or the human spirit. You need to have heart and passion to get in the ring and go for twelve rounds. If you don't believe in anything and you don't have any inner place to go when you need that extra push, you won't be able to finish the match, no matter what condition you're in.

When Hilary Swank trained at Gleason's, she'd bring her dog. She fought for him. Who or what do you fight for?

— COACH'S CORNER —

You have to believe.
If you don't believe, you'll go nowhere.

# Boxing's Mental Benefits

After doing the month-long Gleason's training program, your body will show boxing's benefits. You'll lose weight. You'll feel stronger. You'll get that sexy line down the center of your abs and sides of your thighs. You'll sleep better and feel more energized.

And while it's more difficult to quantify the mental changes you'll see, they will make an even bigger impact on your day-to-day life. Once you start boxing, you will feel your confidence rise. The satisfaction of powering through a tough workout makes you believe in your own strength, stamina, devotion, and willpower. You may surprise yourself and discover a side to you that you didn't know existed. Because our program will increase your strength and fitness, you may notice a little swagger in your step. Maybe you'll even run up the steps two at a time just because you can. Knowing that you can defend yourself may make you feel bolder and more sure of yourself. Everybody takes away different things from boxing.

## Self-confidence

"I've learned that I can keep going much longer than I ever thought I could. Knowing I can push myself, no matter how tired I am, makes me feel more confident."

—JoEllen VanOuwerkerk, age 48

## Calmness

The best boxers have a quiet center, a sense of peace. Too much excitement, or worse, anxiety and nervousness, sap your strength. If you waste your energy by being too jumpy, you can't focus on your goal at hand: to land punches and defend yourself against them. Because boxing demands superfocus, after you begin training, you will become calmer and more centered in all parts of your life.

"I've gained peace of mind from challenging myself, testing my limits, and overcoming my fear." —Emily, age 31

## Anger Release

Any kind of physical exercise, especially a workout as intense as boxing, burns off anger. So if you were motivated to get into the sport to release anger and other bad feelings, it will work and you will feel more satisfied and happier in all areas of your life. Plus, once you get into the sport, you will see that anger and boxing don't mix. Angry boxers are not winning boxers. If a boxer is angry, she's not focusing and is wild and out of control. In fact, a good strategy is to make your opponent angry so that she drops her arms, lunges, telegraphs her moves, wastes her energy, and forgets her strategy.

"I'm now comfortable in my own skin and have a great body image because my perception has shifted. It's no longer important to me to be thin or look a certain way; instead, it's important to be strong and for my body to function at a high level. Also, I rarely feel angry or aggressive out in the world because I've found a specific focus for that kind of energy and emotion."

—Golden Gloves winner Geneve Brossard, age 28

## Pride

Once you learn the skill of boxing and build your strength and stamina, you will feel proud of yourself. And you should: Boxing is a tough sport, so if you stick with your training and master the moves, you should feel good about yourself. People who are proud of their accomplishments stand up for themselves and don't take mess from anybody. They are strong and strong-willed and feel good about themselves, backed by the self-respect that they have earned through the sport.

"I feel proud of my accomplishments and hold them close to me whenever I doubt myself. I don't even need to talk about my boxing to feel good. It gives me a private source of self-confidence."

—Golden Gloves winner Ruth O'Sullivan, age 29

## Positive Outlook

Negativity is the sign of a loser, so we don't see much of that at Gleason's. People who want to become boxers have a positive outlook on life. They believe they are winners, and the sport, when done correctly, encourages these feelings. Working out—and working out hard—lifts the spirits. Performing well lifts them even more.

"I let off all my steam when I train, so I can go home to my husband and kids with a calm disposition and a positive outlook."

—Lawson, age 39

## Concentration

Boxing hones concentration. The best boxers come into the gym with clear minds and are driven and focused while training and while fighting. A good fighter can't be distracted by anything—the crowd, her opponent, her fear, or even her trainer. She has to be focused on her form, moves, and strategies. Because boxing demands total concentration, the ability to focus spills over into the rest of her life. She finds herself able to shut out the distractions of the world, and even the noise in her head, so that she can focus on what's most important to her at the moment.

"Boxing has helped me focus more in school, at work, and in my personal life."                                                    —Maureen Shea, 24

## Parting Shots

Despite all of the strength, skill, and stamina that boxing involves, when it comes down to it, it is a mental sport, a mind game. In the ring, don't bet on the fighter with the hardest punch or the fastest moves. Put your money on the competitor who is smart, focused, driven, and strategic. This is particularly true near the end of the fight: Once your physical stamina sputters out, the mental edge makes the difference between winner and loser.

For you, your mind is the key to success with this program. To be a fighter and to make it through demanding workouts, you will have to use your mind to focus; learn punches, moves, and strategies; push away any negative thoughts; and power through fatigue. If you do this, you will see a payoff, and you will see it right away: Physically, you will have a new body—stronger, sleeker, faster, and more fit. And you will also have a new mind: Your concentration will increase; you will feel happier, more confident, and relaxed.

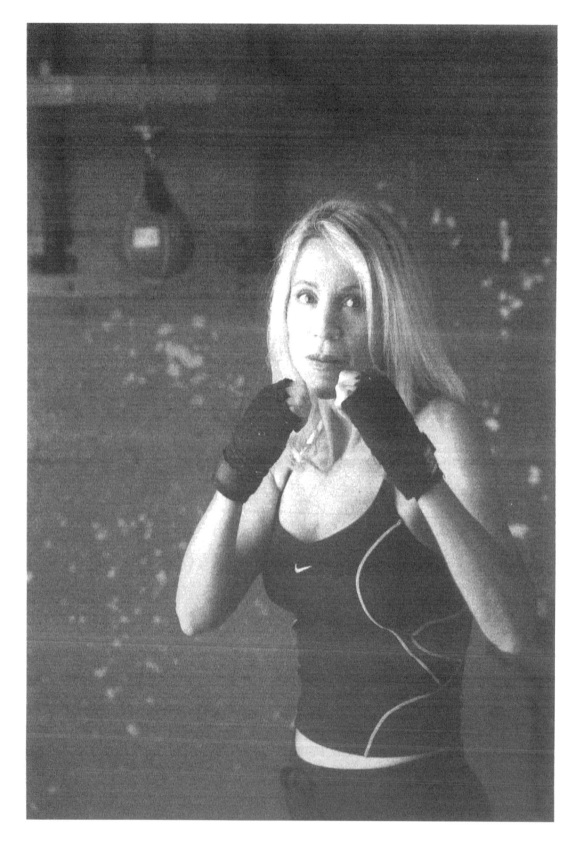

# 3
# Live Right

Eating nutritious food, drinking plenty of water, listening to your body, and getting enough rest are the cornerstones of good health—and your boxing workout won't work out unless you pay attention to these cornerstones. You should be just as disciplined about taking care of your body, including being careful about what you eat and drink and how much sleep you get—as you are about your mental focus, your boxing skills, and your physical fitness. Once you begin training, you'll notice that you feel more energetic, stronger, leaner, and healthier, and you'll want to take even better care of yourself. As you begin to take better care of your body as a whole, you'll be able to box longer and harder and see and feel the results more quickly.

## — COACH'S CORNER —

To start boxing, you have to be clean. You have to live right.

## ★ WHAT THE DOCTOR ORDERS ★

Part of staying healthy means getting a yearly checkup with a health professional, including tests and screenings. Before you start this program, make sure you've got a clean bill of health from your doctor. And if you have a health problem or you're a beginning exerciser with a low level of fitness, check with your doctor to make sure this program is right for you.

## What to Eat

At Gleason's we don't recommend a specific eating plan. There is no one "boxing diet." Everybody has different needs. But just like in every other aspect of our training philosophy, we are old school, straightforward, and stick to the basics. Eating doesn't have to be complicated. Diet rules and gimmicks don't work for everyone—and often they don't work at all, so we don't pay attention to them. So keep it simple and follow common sense guidelines: If you want to have a lean boxer's body, feel strong and healthy, maximize your workouts, and consume a balanced mix of foods. Figure out the kinds of foods that are good for you and that you like and fit the way you live. We don't want you to deny yourself; we just want you to be smart. If you want a cookie, eat one, but don't consume the whole bag. If you want a steak, go ahead and have a four-ounce steak, but not the whole cow, not every day, and not too close to the workout when you won't have time to digest it. If your goal is both fitness and weight loss, watching what you eat is critical. So be practical and understand these basic facts about nutrition:

◆ Protein will help you build muscle. Each fish, poultry, lean red meat (if you're a meat-eater), or tofu once or twice a day, and broil or bake rather than fry. Nuts and beans also contain plenty of protein, so eat these between one and three times a day. Eggs are high in protein, but the yolks contain cholesterol, which raises your risk of heart disease. So eat them in moderation or consume the whites only. Dairy products like cheese and milk are high in protein, but choose low-fat options and avoid consuming them too close to your workout, particularly if you have trouble digesting milk products.

◆ Eat as many vegetables as you like. Leafy greens like lettuce, broccoli, spinach, kale, and collard greens provide the most vitamins and other health benefits. It is best to steam them and avoid heavy sauces or too much butter, which pile on calories, reduce nutritional value, and sometimes prove difficult to digest.

◆ Try to include whole-grain foods at every meal. Whole grains are easy to digest and provide quick, healthy energy. It's probably easiest at breakfast time, since so many ready-to-eat cereals—hot and cold—contain bran, whole wheat, oats, and cornmeal. Avoid sugary, highly-processed brands, consume them with low-fat or skim milk, and don't add extra sugar. Also, if bran and other high-fiber foods make your stools loose, don't eat them too close to your workout for obvious reasons. Other healthy whole grains include brown and wild rice, barley, and bulgur. Read labels carefully and choose whole-grain breads, tortillas, crackers, and muffins.

◆ Eat fruit two or three times a day. Fresh fruit contains plenty of vitamins, water, and few calories and, for most people, is easy to digest. Fruits like apples, melon, pears, grapes, and cherries, contain "natural" sugars, which equal quick energy in a healthy package.

◆ Keep an eye on carbohydrates without being fanatical. Eat white foods—rice, bread, pasta, potatoes—sparingly, since their nutritional value is low. However, because carbohydrates are easy to digest, which is important when you're working out, don't eliminate them altogether. Instead choose whole-grain pasta, brown or wild rice, and whole-wheat bread.

◆ Avoid sugar, including sugary drinks. Turn away from candy, desserts, and soda as an energy fix. Although sugar—or simple carbohydrates—do provide quick energy, they contain only empty calories. Plus the rush doesn't last and can turn into a crash. While you don't have to deprive yourself, keep sugar to a minimum and read labels carefully to avoid hidden sugars in soft drinks and processed foods.

✦ Choose fats wisely. Stay away from saturated fats found in processed foods, fatty red meats, and butter. Also keep fried foods to a minimum because they are high in calories and can make you feel "heavy" before a workout—and after, too. Instead, sauté or broil foods in plant oils like olive, canola, soy, and sunflower.

## — COACH'S CORNER —

The best food in the world for boxing: rice and beans. It's simple, it's not expensive, it's not heavy, and it tastes good. Hint: Substitute brown rice for white rice.

## ★ WHEN TO EAT ★

Timing your meals and snacks is a balancing act, particularly with boxing: If you eat too much, too close to your workout, you'll feel bloated, slow, and even ill. But if you don't eat at all or enough, you'll be weak and lightheaded. It's best to pay attention to your own body and digestion, but as a rule of thumb, eat a large meal at least three hours before your workout. Time a small meal for one or two hours before exercising. Some people can eat while they workout; do what feels right for you.

# ★ LOSING IT ★

Boxing is a sport of weight classes, so we understand the importance of how much you weigh. But don't be obsessed with weight. If weight loss is your goal, you will lose weight with our program as long as you don't gorge yourself after your workout. Boxing is hard work, and a 130-pound. amateur boxer burns more than 700 calories during a fight. Shadowboxing, which is the basis of our workout, burns about 530 calories an hour—about the same as running an eleven-minute mile, more than an hour-long high-impact aerobics class, and about twice as much as a brisk walk. If you work out hard and watch what you eat, you will lose weight, but the catch is that exercising hard will make you hungry. So if you want to get fit, strong, and knock off some pounds, follow these tips:

1. Balance eating too much with eating too little. You will feel hungry after your workouts. But be careful not to eat too much—or fatty, sugary foods, which will decrease the weight loss benefits of your workout. Yet, don't restrict calories too much or you'll be too weak to exercise effectively. Balanced and small portions that include lots of fruit, vegetables, and whole grains are key.

2. Eat breakfast. If you skip it—or any meal for that matter—you'll be hungrier later, which may lead to overeating or poor food choices later in the day. If you plan to exercise in the morning, eat a small portion of a food that's easy to digest, like fruit or whole grain.

3. Don't wait too long after exercising to eat. Otherwise, you'll be ravenous, which can lead to binge eating later on. Also, be careful not to eat too fast, or you may end up rushing through your meal and heading back for seconds.

4. Consume energy bars or replacement drinks carefully. Of course, they'll do in an absolute pinch, but most contain large amounts of sugar (and calories) and little or no fiber.

# Water, Water, and More Water

You probably know the rule of thumb: Drink eight glasses or water per day. But when you train, you need to drink much more. Water carries nutrients to the cells and removes waste from them. It also replaces the fluids you "sweat off" during exercise and helps your body regulate your temperature. If you don't drink enough fluids during exercise, you can become dehydrated, particularly in hot, humid weather. In fact, recent reports have shown that not drinking enough fluid can be dangerous, even deadly, for avid exercisers.

Although it may feel like much more, you will lose about one to two liters of water every hour of your boxing workout. You'll need to consume about five to eight ounces of water every fifteen minutes, so keep a glass or bottle of water on hand. Drink as close to the start of your workout as you can without feeling sick and during (sip, so you don't get "water-logged") and after training. Studies show that it's not enough to rely on thirst to tell you when you need to hydrate. Be on the safe side: Keep sipping. A sure way to know if you're getting enough fluids is to check your urine. It should be pale yellow. If it looks darker or heavier, drink more.

For maximum hydration, plain old water is your best option, particularly if you're hoping to lose weight. Sports beverages add electrolytes and minerals that you lose when you sweat. But they also add sugar, calories, and cost. Avoid carbonated soft drinks and milk before you work out. If you need an extra boost, fruit juice may be a good option, but, again, keep an eye on calories. In general, don't drink coffee, tea, and other caffeinated beverages too close to working out. Although caffeine provides a quick hit of "energy," it actually dehydrates you.

In general, as part of an overall plan for good health—and no matter what the beer commercials say—keep alcohol consumption to a minimum.

# A.M. or P.M.: When's the Best Time to Work Out?

The quick answer is any time you want. However, scientific studies have found that the ideal time to exercise is late afternoon/early evening, between 4:00 P.M. and 7:00 P.M. For most of us, hormone levels peak around 6:00 P.M., and other exercise functions are also at their best during this time period.

However, the best way to choose a time to get in your workout depends more on you than on research. Plus, you can also mix it up depending on your schedule. Below, check out the facts about each time of day as you select the best time for you.

## Morning

Of course, this is a great option if you're a morning person who feels energetic in the early hours of the day. Many boxers feel at their best in the early morning; in fact, it's not unusual to find a full house at Gleason's between 7:00 A.M. and 9:00 A.M. It's easier to work out consistently if you do it first thing in the morning—which may be your only free time if you've got a very busy schedule. Exercising in the morning also boosts your energy—and metabolism—for several hours after you've worked out, and the focus that boxing requires will help jumpstart your day. Plus, once your exercise session is under your belt, you'll feel good about yourself. If you choose to work out in the morning, remember that your muscles may be cold and stiff just after you roll out of bed, so do a little extra warming up and stretching.

## Lunchtime

If your work schedule allows and you've got the space, train at lunch. A lunchtime workout is a great stress reliever and will help boost your energy and mental sharpness in the afternoon, when you may be looking for a latte to give you a boost. If noontime works best for you, do your best to avoid letting distractions at work get in the way of your fitness commitment.

## Early to Late Afternoon and Evening

This may be the only time of day you can fit in your workout, particularly if you're really not a morning person. Because your body is, scientifically speaking, at its best at this time, you may find that you can work out harder and longer between 4:00 P.M. and 7:00 P.M. Plus, nearer to the end of the day, your muscles will be warm and loose, and a training session will help relieve the stresses that have built up during the day. However, exercising too close to bedtime can keep you up at night, so be sure to schedule your training session one to three hours before you plan to go to sleep.

# Parting Shots

Diet is part of mental discipline. A boxer has to have a mind like steel and a body like iron, but you can't build a body that strong or a mind that sharp if you don't take care of yourself. Every day boxers who stay up late every night and seem to eat nothing but fast food and drink little other than soda come into our gym. And sometimes they are successful on hard work and sheer talent alone. But that's rare. People who don't have the good sense to take care of their bodies rarely go the distance. Plus, we've seen it happen time and again: Once you start training, you won't want to put any crap into your body. You'll see that your body can look and feel good, so you'll want to keep it as healthy as possible to perform at your peak. We're not going to tell you step-by-step what to eat, what to drink, and what to do with your free time. It's on you. All we can do is remind you to be smart and practical and take great care of yourself.

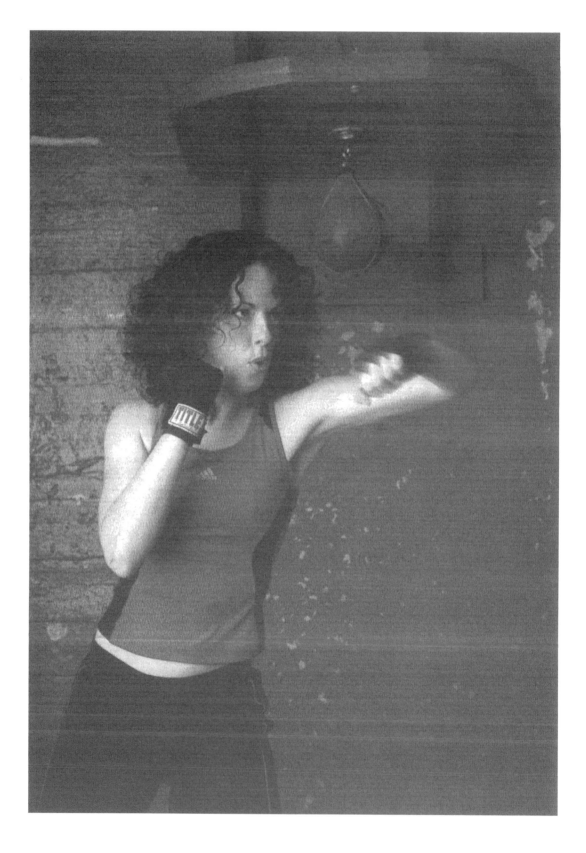

# 4

# Boxing Basics

**N**ow that you've learned how to think like a boxer, it's time to learn how to move like one. In this chapter, you'll learn how to stand, punch, and, most importantly, defend yourself.

Unlike those cardioboxing classes offered at your gym, we want you to concentrate on the quality of your form, not the quantity of your punches. First, you need to master the technique. Soon enough, you'll be able to rip off highly effective, rapid-fire combinations. But for now, go slow, pay attention to every part of your body to make sure your form is correct, and do your moves over and over. The proper form should be a reflex, and it will only become second nature to you if you practice. At Gleason's Gym, there's no faking good form so you have to constantly be real with yourself. You're learning how to box *for real*. We're getting you ready to fight, not to bounce around some aerobics studio. If you don't have the proper form to back you up, you'll go down fast.

Before you begin to practice all of the boxing basics outlined in this chapter, clear out a space in front of the biggest mirror you can find. If you were at Gleason's in Brooklyn, we'd grab your arms and put them in position. We'd poke your stomach to make sure it's pulled in properly or punch your sides to show you that you've dropped your arms and left yourself vulnerable. The boxers training around you would yell instructions. But in your own home, it's up to you to check your own form every step of the way—and watching yourself in a mirror is the best way to do that. We'll tell you everything you need to know, but it's up to you to listen and take responsibility for yourself. Remember, a smaller boxer with good technique and good footing will always beat a larger, more powerful opponent who doesn't have technique. The sweet secret is that it is all about *style.*

## ★ ADVICE TO THE NEWBIE BOXER ★

*Since you can't join us at the gym,*
*our fighters want to share their best pointers*
*for you newbies who are just starting out.*

"Don't worry about looking stupid. No one is judging you. Move your head. Just go with the flow. It's [okay] to feel overwhelmed in the beginning."                           —Golden Gloves winner Geneve Brossard, age 28

"Don't get discouraged because some combination you're learning flies right out the window when you're boxing. When you're nervous and trying to defend yourself, you tend to keep repeating what you know instead of forcing yourself to try something new. Try to forget your ego to look good in the ring, and practice something new to improve your repertoire."                                            —JoEllen VanOuwerkerk, age 48

"Be honest with yourself when you're training. Don't ever underestimate your opponent. And listen only to your trainer. You need to trust him 150 percent."                                                  —Maureen Shea, age 24

"Be patient with yourself."                                    —Angela, age 31

"The mental part is the hardest part. Set some concrete goals to build your confidence and then start to vary them. Also, don't feel self-conscious when you're shadowboxing."                    —Emily, age 31

"Focus on your technique in the beginning—aligning your punches and getting your footwork right. And make sure you get enough sleep; your body will reward you for it."

—Golden Gloves winner Ruth O'Sullivan, age 29

"Don't get frustrated; give yourself permission to make a lot of mistakes. And do it at least three times a week for best results."    —Lawson, age 39

## ★ ARE YOU A SOUTHPAW? ★

*What You Need to Know*

A southpaw is simply a left-handed boxer. Since most boxers fight right-handed (aka orthodox), every move described in this book is tailored to the orthodox stance, but southpaws stand differently, throw punches in the opposite direction, and block punches in the opposite direction. So if you're a southpaw, simply reverse sides. For instance, you'll throw your jab with your right hand, rather than your left. Even if you're not a southpaw by nature, it pays to train as one, once you master your basic skills. (You'll do it in Week Four.) Many fighters are thrown off by southpaws, which offers a natural advantage to the left-handed competitor. In fact, some professional boxers refuse to fight against southpaws in early rounds because they don't feel prepared to fight a lefty. If you can switch stances, not only will it make for a more challenging, interesting, well-rounded workout, you'll also win a lot of fights, too.

# On Your Feet

How you stand and move in the ring is the difference between winning or losing a fight. You don't want to just stand there like you have lead in your pants. With heavy, flat feet, it's impossible to defend yourself against any type of punch. Defense is the *key* to your offense. If you defend yourself well, you sap your opponent's strength and make her waste her energy, which is a great way to win a fight and save your face. Plus, it's always better to hit than to be hit.

Try moving from one foot to the other, following one foot behind the other, not side to side. It allows you to shift your body weight sequentially. When you place your weight on one foot, you can pivot off it to get all your body torque into the punch.

Make sure your weight is evenly distributed. You do not want to lean forward because you can get off balance and fall forward or walk into a punch.

# Stance: The Snake

## GOAL

This is your basic fighting position, the foundation of boxing. You should always be in this position, unless you're in the middle of a punch. Your hands protect your face, your forearms protect your stomach, your shoulders protect your chin, and your body becomes the smallest possible target, which means that there is less of you to punch. Also, the snake stance allows you to put your whole body behind each punch—from the balls of your feet, through your legs, midsection, shoulders, and finally your arms and fist. This is more effective than standing upright and punching with only your arms. At first, you may find this position awkward, and you may have trouble keeping your arms up and elbows tucked into your sides. But as you get stronger and practice the position correctly, this stance will become very natural to you.

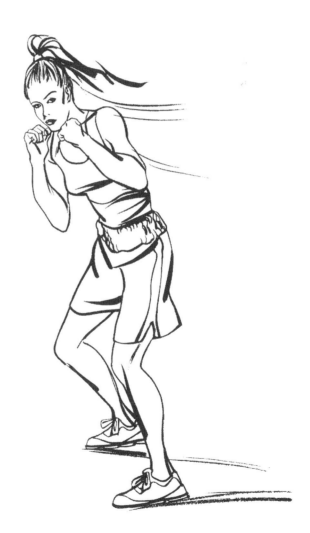

**STEPS**

1. Stand with feet shoulder-width apart, your right foot about 18-inches behind the left, right toe pointed out at slightly wider than a 45-degree angle. Point your left toe forward, turned slightly inward.
2. Keep your legs almost straight and your weight centered, and pull your bellybutton in toward your spine.
3. Raise both fists to chin level, palms facing inward with your elbows tight to your sides to protect your ribs.
4. Tuck your chin toward your chest, and direct your gaze forward at your target, like you're looking through your eyebrows.

**FOCUS**

Think of yourself as a king cobra, coiled at the bottom with your neck and head weaving around your opponent, ready to strike at any time.

**ALWAYS**

◆ Keep your weight on the balls of your feet, so you can easily shuffle around the ring. You never want to be caught flat-footed.

◆ Keep your fists at chin-height with your elbows tucked, so your head and body are always protected. At Gleason's if we see a boxer with her elbows up, we give her a punch in the side to remind her that she's leaving herself wide open.

◆ Make your target area as small as possible.

**NEVER**

◆ Drop your hands or allow your elbows to come away from your ribcage, or you will get punched in your side.

◆ Lean forward, or you'll get punched in the nose.

◆ Lean backward, or you'll lose your balance and get knocked down.

**VARIATION**

If you are a southpaw, your feet and shoulders should be in the reverse position. That is, your right foot and shoulder will lead, and your left foot and shoulder will be furthest from your opponent. Southpaws should always reverse the hands and feet positions from here on out.

## HOW TO MOVE

When you're in the ring, you should *always* be moving. It'll make it harder for your opponent to hit you and easier for you to hit her because she'll never know where you're going. That means footwork is key to winning a fight. You shouldn't have to think about your footwork; if you're spending too much time worrying about what your feet are doing, you'll lose focus and get beaten. So how you move in the ring should be as natural as walking down the street. But you'll only master your footwork by learning to do it correctly and then practicing it.

There are five ways to move in the ring:

1. Toward your opponent, which is called advancing
2. Away from your opponent, which is called retreating
3. To the left
4. To the right
5. In a circle around your opponent, either clockwise or counterclockwise

We're going to give you two drills straight away to help you practice your footwork. Start slowly, and only after you nail the form, try it again with more speed.

# Do This Drill: Run the Cross

## GOAL

This left-right-advance-retreat drill, designed to help you master your movement, will teach you to float around the ring with speed and agility.

**STEPS**

1. Start in snake position with your weight centered. Shuffle to the left by taking a small step with your left (front) foot, followed by your right (back) foot. Repeat 3 times.
2. Shuffle back to the right, stepping first with your right (back) foot and then your left (front) foot. Repeat 3 times, which brings you back to where you started.
3. Advance toward your (real or imaginary) opponent by stepping forward first with your left (front) foot and quickly following with your right (back) foot. Repeat 3 times.
4. Retreat by stepping back first with your right (back) foot and then your left (front) foot. Repeat 3 times, until you return to your starting position.
5. Repeat the entire sequence 5 more times, and then switch the order. Move right, left, retreat, and advance. Repeat 5 times. Change order and repeat.

**FOCUS**

Be light-footed. The ability to move around swiftly is the key to winning matches.

**ALWAYS**

- Hold your snake position.
- Avoid being flat-footed no matter how tired you are. Your body weight should remain on the balls of your feet, never on your heels.
- Lead with the foot closest to the direction in which you want to go.
- Keep your abs pulled in tight.

**NEVER**

- Hop, skip, jump, or gallop. You always want at least one foot firmly planted on the floor.
- Cross your feet over each other, or you'll trip.
- Turn your back to your opponent.
- Lean. Not only will you be off-balance, but you'll also give your opponent a clue as to where you're going. Think snake position.

# Do This Drill: The Circle

## GOAL

Fights take place in a square that is called a ring. It doesn't sound like it makes sense, but it does. During a match, boxers move in a circle. You never want your opponent to know where you're going. Moving around her in a circle, clockwise or counterclockwise, opens her up to more powerful punches, like a left hook. If she is flat-footed and you circle her, she won't even see your glove coming for her head and then it's lights out.

## STEPS

1. Recruit either a friend, who will stand still for you for two minutes, or a chair. Either will work just fine. No, you're not going to hit her!

2. Assume the snake position and face your opponent (your pal or the chair).

3. Begin to circle clockwise by stepping to the left with your left (front) foot and following with your right (back) foot. Be careful not to cross your feet because you will be off- balance. The motion is more like a shuffle.

4. Continue slowly around your opponent until you're back to your starting position.

5. Switch directions by stepping to the right with your right (back) foot, followed by your left (front) foot. Go around twice. Switch direction and repeat. Switch direction and repeat again.

## FOCUS

Concentrate on remaining in the perfect snake position throughout the entire circle. Your left shoulder (or if you're a southpaw, your right shoulder) should always be facing your opponent.

## ALWAYS

♦ Face your opponent in the snake stance. When circling your opponent, it's very easy to fall out of position. Your shoulders should never be square with your opponent's; that opens up your head and body for punches.

♦ Make sure your back foot stays behind you and pointed out, not next to your front foot and pointed toward your opponent. You need it behind you to stay balanced and to remain as small a target as possible.

NEVER

♦ Hop. It may be your instinct to start galloping around your opponent because it's faster, but you never want to let both feet leave the mat at the same time. If you're hit, you'll go sailing.

♦ Square off your shoulders to your opponent.

♦ Take your eyes off of your target.

♦ Drop your hands.

# How to Punch

There are four basic types of punches in boxing: the jab, the straight right (or straight left, if you're a southpaw), the hook, and the uppercut. As you learn them, move slowly and concentrate on your technique. Power punches without proper form just look desperate and sloppy, and they'll sap your energy. Graceful punches with the proper form will accumulate power en route to your target and require less effort on your part. That means you can last longer and punch harder.

Before you throw your first punch, it's important to learn how to make a proper fist, so you don't hurt your hand.

# How to Make a Fist

## GOAL

Turn your hand into a weapon and be able to sustain impact without injury.

**STEPS**

1. Curl your fingers into your palm.
2. Wrap your thumb around the outside of your fingers, so your thumb knuckle rests on your middle finger, between its top and middle knuckle.

**FOCUS**

The long section of your fingers should form a flat plane. When you punch, concentrate on making contact with your target with *all* four knuckles.

**ALWAYS**

◆ Keep your thumb outside of your fingers.

◆ Strike with your top knuckles, not your fingers.

**NEVER**

◆ Aim to strike with your outside (pinky) knuckles because they tend to break more easily.

# The Left Jab

## GOAL

A speedy punch powered from your shoulder, the left jab is your bread-and-butter punch, the one you will use most often. Not only does it make for an excellent defense, but it also helps knock your opponent off balance. The other purpose of the jab is to occupy your opponent's mind (and her eyes), so you can set up for more powerful combinations. Remember, a boxer with no jab is no good, so really concentrate on your form.

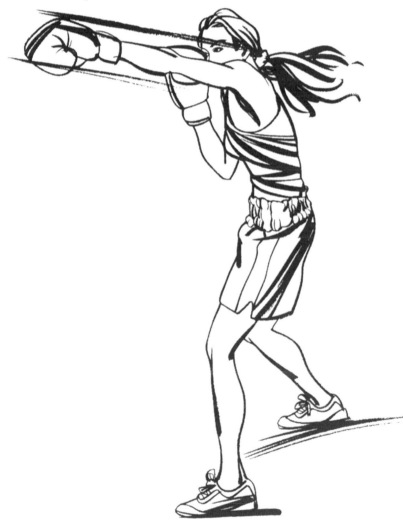

1. Starting in snake position, step forward with your left foot and at the same time extend your left arm, from the shoulder. Aim for the spot between your opponent's chin and chest.

2. During the final third of the extension, rotate your fist so your closed palm is facing down. This twist at the end is what gives your punch power and also protects your wrist.

3. Bring your arm back quickly and get back into the snake position by reversing through the same exact motion. This may feel complicated and awkward at first, particularly because you may not be used to twisting your wrist at the end of the punch, but just practice it.

FOCUS

Remember this should be one smooth, fluid motion. At first, just get the rhythm of the movement by thinking snake, step, arm, snap, step, snake. Put some force behind it by imagining your arm as a screw, rotating *through* your target.

ALWAYS

◆ Keep your jabs swift and sharp by snapping your fist just before impact.

◆ Step forward as you jab to help prevent overreaching. If you just punch with only your arm, you won't have as much power—or balance—than if you step into the punch.

◆ Maintain your balance throughout the punch by keeping your weight equally distributed between your feet.

NEVER

◆ Use a pushing movement to deliver a jab. Don't paw your opponent—punch her. Your fist should always follow a smooth screwing motion.

◆ Rush your technique. Practice your jabs in slow motion until you master the movement.

◆ Aim for your opponent's forehead. If she moves one inch, you'll miss, causing you to get out of position and lose your balance. Then you'll get hit.

# Jab to the Body

## GOAL

Another speedy punch, powered from your shoulder. This punch is a variation of the left jab and targets the midsection of your opponent's body. It also serves as an excellent defense, and it can help knock your opponent off balance. The other purpose of the jab is to occupy your opponent's mind (and her eyes), so you can set up for more powerful combinations. Remember, a boxer with no jab is no good, so really concentrate on your form.

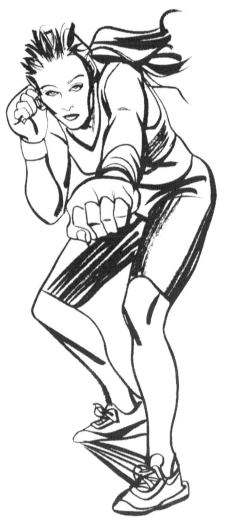

1. Starting in snake position, step forward with your left foot, bend your knees, and at the same time extend your left arm, from the shoulder. While you'll aim most jabs for your opponent's neck, you can hit your opponent with a jab anywhere on her body as long as you're within striking distance. Remember, to deliver a jab to the body, aim lower by bending your knees.

2. During the final third of the extension, rotate your fist so your closed palm is facing down. This twist at the end is what gives your punch power and also protects your wrist.

3. Bring your arm back quickly and get back into the snake position, by reversing through the same exact motion. This may feel complicated and awkward at first, particularly because you may not be used to twisting your wrist at the end of the punch, but just practice it.

**FOCUS**

Remember this should be one smooth, fluid motion. At first, just get the rhythm of the movement by thinking snake, step, arm, snap, step, snake. Put some force behind it by imagining your arm as a screw, rotating *through* your target.

**ALWAYS**

- Keep your jabs swift and sharp by snapping your fist just before impact.
- Step forward as you jab to help prevent overreaching. If you just punch with only your arm, you won't have as much power—or balance—than if you step into the punch.
- Maintain your balance throughout the punch by keeping your weight equally distributed between your feet.
- Remember to keep your torso upright, rather than leaning forward.

**NEVER**

- Use a pushing movement to deliver a jab. Don't paw your opponent—punch her. Your fist should always follow a smooth screwing motion.
- Rush your technique. Practice your jabs in slow motion until you master the movement.

# The Straight Right

## GOAL

This is your money shot, the one most likely to knock out your opponent. If you do it correctly, you'll use the pivot to power the punch, which means that you're combining the power of your arm, shoulder, and thigh. The catch is that it takes longer for your right fist to reach your opponent's body because it has farther to travel, and if you miss, any experienced boxer will be able to nail you for it.

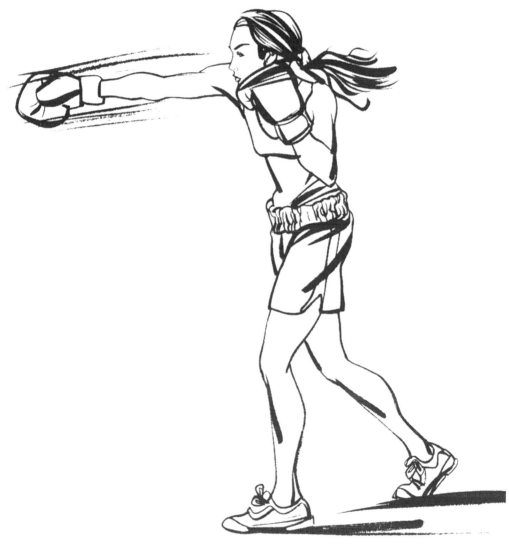

1. Shift your weight to your front foot and pivot off your back foot, rotating through your hips as you extend your right arm toward the point between your opponent's chin, neck, and chest. Keep your eyes focused there.

2. As your body weight shifts forward, snap your wrist so your fist quickly turns palm down and punch through your target.

3. Retract your fist, retracing your motion until you return to your starting position.

FOCUS

While the power of the jab comes from your shoulder, the power of the right cross originates in your hips. Picture your body whipping around, allowing your right fist to pick up speed as it moves forward.

ALWAYS

◆ Power this punch by turning from your hips through your core.
◆ Keep your left hand by your chin to guard your face.
◆ Keep your left foot planted so that you stay balanced.

NEVER

◆ Rely on the straight right as your main form of attack. It takes too long to deliver and opens you up for a counterpunch.
◆ Whip your entire body around because it'll cause you to overreach and lose balance. Only turn your hips. Your power comes from the hips and shoulders.

# Straight Right to the Body

## GOAL

This is the punch that'll knock the wind out of your opponent if you land it successfully in her stomach or ribs. It'll take her a beat to recover, and in the meantime you can deliver a few combinations that will bring the match to an early end. If you do it correctly, you'll use the pivot to power the punch, which means that you're combining the power of your arm, shoulder, and thigh. The catch is that it takes longer for your right fist to reach your opponent's body, because it has farther to travel, and if you miss, any experienced boxer will be able to nail you for it.

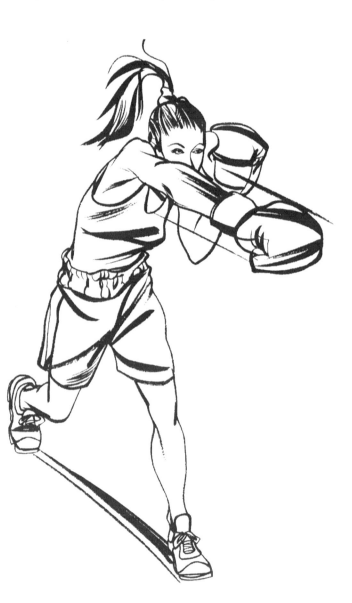

1. Keeping your torso in snake position, squat down by bending your knees until your shoulders come in line with your target. Shift your weight to your front foot and pivot off your back foot, rotating through your hips as you extend your right arm toward your opponent's midsection. Using the force of your rotating hips and your shoulders, drive your punch through your opponent's body.
2. As your body weight shifts forward, snap your wrist so your fist quickly turns palm down and punch through your target.
3. Retract your fist, retracing your motion, until you return to your starting position.

FOCUS    While the power of the jab comes from your shoulder, the power of the straight right originates in your hips. Picture your body whipping around, allowing your right fist to pick up speed as it moves forward.

ALWAYS
- Power this punch by turning from your hips through your core.
- Keep your left hand by your chin to guard your face.
- Keep your left foot planted so that you stay balanced.

NEVER
- Rely on the straight right as your main form of attack. It takes too long to deliver and opens you up for a counterpunch.
- Whip your entire body around because it'll cause you to overreach and lose balance. Only turn your hips. Your power comes from the hips and shoulders.

# Right Overhand

## GOAL

This power punch is similar to the straight right. The only difference is that your fist moves downward rather than parallel to the floor. Pull this punch out if your opponent is short or squatting.

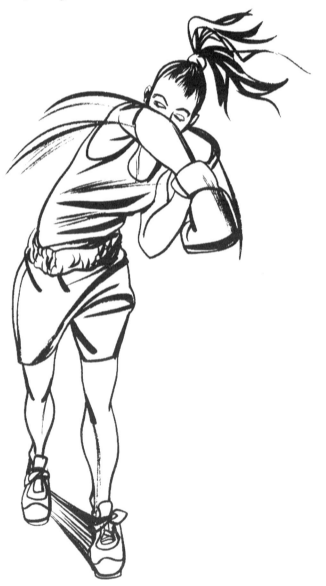

1. Keeping your torso in snake position, squat down by bending your knees until your shoulders come in line with your target. Shift your weight to your front foot and pivot off your back foot, rotating through your hips as you extend your right arm toward your opponent's midsection. Using the force of your rotating hips and your shoulders, drive your punch down through your opponent's body.

2. As your body weight shifts forward, snap your wrist so your fist quickly turns palm down and punch through your target.

3. Retract your fist, retracing your motion, until you return to starting position.

**FOCUS**

While the power of the jab comes from your shoulder, the power of the right overhand originates in your hips. Picture your body whipping around, allowing your right fist to pick up speed as it moves forward.

**ALWAYS**

◆ Power this punch by turning from your hips through your core.

◆ Keep your left hand by your chin to guard your face.

◆ Keep your left foot planted so that you stay balanced.

**NEVER**

◆ Rely on the right overhand as your main form of attack. It takes too long to deliver and opens you up for a counterpunch.

◆ Whip your entire body around because it'll cause you to overreach and lose balance. Only turn your hips. Your power comes from the hips and shoulders.

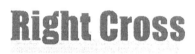

# Right Cross

## GOAL

This variation is the same as a straight right, only you're punching *across* your opponent's chin rather than straight into it.

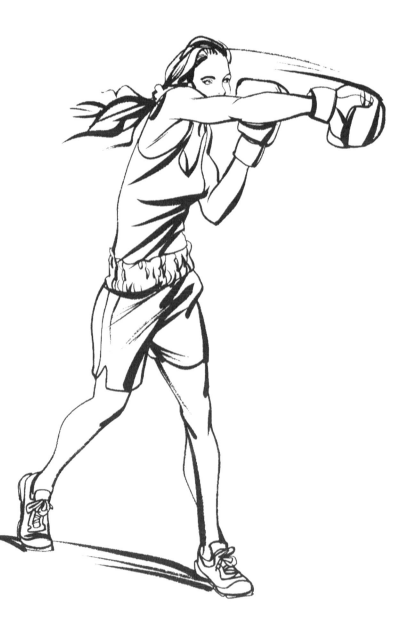

**STEPS**

1. Keeping your torso in snake position, squat down by bending your knees until your shoulders come in line with your target. Shift your weight to your front foot and pivot off your back foot, rotating through your hips as you extend your right arm toward your opponent's chin. Using the force of your rotating hips and your shoulders, drive your punch across your opponent's chin.

2. As your body weight shifts forward, snap your wrist so your fist quickly turns palm down and punch through your target.

3. Retract your fist, retracing your motion, until you return to your starting position.

**FOCUS**

While the power of the jab comes from your shoulder, the power of the right cross originates in your hips. Picture your body whipping around, allowing your right fist to pick up speed as it moves forward.

**ALWAYS**

◆ Power this punch by turning from your hips through your core.

◆ Keep your left hand by your chin to guard your face.

◆ Keep your left foot planted so that you stay balanced.

**NEVER**

◆ Rely on the right cross as your main form of attack. It takes too long to deliver and opens you up for a counterpunch.

◆ Whip your entire body around because it'll cause you to overreach and lose balance. Only turn your hips. Your power comes from the hips and shoulders.

# The Left Hook

## GOAL

The left hook is your finale punch. Not only will you use it to finish many combinations, but also if delivered correctly, this is the punch that'll blindside your opponent and take her down. She'll never even see it coming, since it hooks around, outside of her line of vision. If your left hook is good, you're gold.

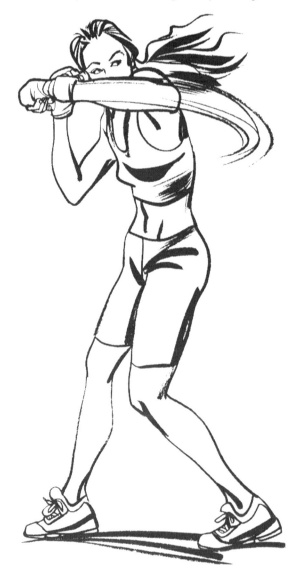

1. Start in snake position. Shift your weight onto your right (back) foot.
2. Leading with your fist, raise your left elbow, so your upper arm is parallel to the floor and forms a right angle with your forearm.
3. To deliver the blow, rotate your hips to the right, pivoting the ball of your left (front) foot to the right, and follow through with your fist, thumb down, aiming for your opponent's shoulder.

FOCUS

While the power of the jab comes from your shoulder, the power of the left hook originates in your hips. Picture your body whipping around, allowing your left fist to pick up speed as it moves forward.

ALWAYS

◆ Return to the snake position, following the same motion, with a sharp snap.
◆ Keep your right fist up to protect your face.
◆ Keep your left wrist straight and parallel to the floor while punching to prevent injury.

NEVER

◆ Allow your left elbow to drop. Your arm must be parallel to the floor, or your punch will not carry force, or worse, you'll injure your shoulder on impact.
◆ Keep your feet planted. The twisting motion of the left hook is so dramatic that you must pivot your feet so the twist doesn't injure your knees.
◆ Aim for your opponent's forehead. You'll miss if she moves.

# Left Hook to the Body

## GOAL

Embrace the left hook as your finale punch. Not only will you use it to finish many combinations, but also if delivered correctly, this is the punch that'll blindside your opponent. She'll never even see it coming, since it hooks around, outside of her line of vision. When your opponent is jabbing you, this punch makes for a particularly effective response because you can catch her ribs wide open. With this punch, you can take her down.

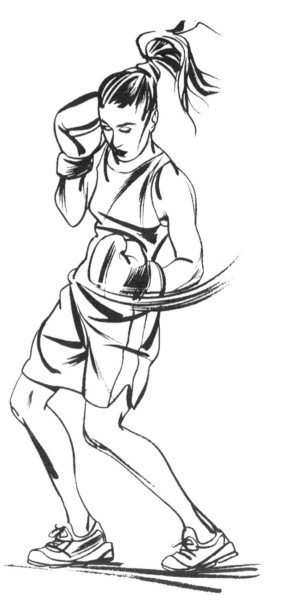

STEPS    1. Start in snake position. Shift your weight onto your right (back) foot.

2. Keeping your torso straight, bend your knees until your shoulders are parallel to your target. When you deliver the blow, keep your left elbow close to your side and punch in and upward, crossing your body. Your palm should be facing you, and your forearm should be at about a 45-degree angle to the floor.

FOCUS    Keep your left elbow close to your side, and whip your hip around behind it to gain force.

ALWAYS   ◆ Return to the snake position, following the same motion, with a sharp snap.

◆ Keep your right fist up to protect your face.

◆ Keep your left wrist straight and parallel to the floor while punching to prevent injury.

NEVER    ◆ Keep your feet planted. The twisting motion of the left hook is so dramatic that you must pivot your feet so the twist doesn't injure your knees.

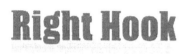

# Right Hook

## GOAL

While left hooks are almost always used as endings to combinations, you can throw a surprise right hook on its own. The form of a right hook is different than that of a left hook.

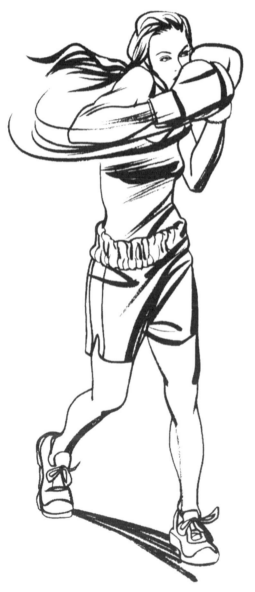

**THE GLEASON'S GYM TOTAL BODY BOXING WORKOUT FOR WOMEN**

1. Raise your right arm so it's parallel with the ground; form a 90-degree angle with your forearm and upper arm.
2. Unlike the motion for the left hook, don't rotate your fist so that your palm is facing down. Instead, keep your palm facing you and your thumb knuckle pointed upward, as if you're about to clink a beer mug. (Keeping your first upright allows you to get the punch off quicker.)
3. Rotate your right hip forward, pivot on the ball of your right foot, and punch through your opponent's shoulder.

**FOCUS**

While the power of the jab comes from your shoulder, the power of the right hook originates in your hips. Picture your body whipping around, allowing your right fist to pick up speed as it moves forward.

**ALWAYS**

◆ Return to the snake position, following the same motion, with a sharp snap.
◆ Keep your left fist up to protect your face.
◆ Keep your right wrist straight and parallel to the floor while punching to prevent injury.

**NEVER**

◆ Keep your feet planted. The twisting motion of the right hook is so dramatic that you must pivot your feet so the twist doesn't injure your knees.

# Right Hook to the Body

## GOAL

The right hook to the body is especially effective when your opponent is on the ropes. She can see the punch coming from a mile away, but she can't go anywhere.

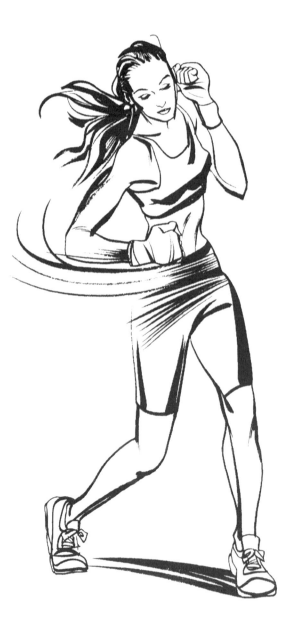

STEPS

1. Raise your right arm so it's parallel with the ground; form a 90-degree angle with your forearm and upper arm.
2. Bend your knees to lower your body.
3. Unlike the motion for the left hook, don't rotate your fist so that your palm is facing down. Instead, keep you palm facing you and your thumb knuckle pointed upward, as if you're about to clink a beer mug. (Keeping your first upright allows you to get the punch off quicker.)
4. Rotate your right hip forward, pivot on the ball of your right foot, and aim your punch toward your opponent's midsection. Remember to keep your thumb up and palm facing you, not facing the floor.

FOCUS

While the power of the jab comes from your shoulder, the power of the right hook to the body originates in your hips. Picture your body whipping around, allowing your right fist to pick up speed as it moves forward.

ALWAYS

◆ Keep your thumb up and palm facing you, not facing the floor.
◆ Keep your left fist up to protect your face.

NEVER

◆ Keep your feet planted. The twisting motion of the right hook is so dramatic that you must pivot your feet so the twist doesn't injure your knees.

# The Right Uppercut

This blow is the punishment for any boxer who leans forward in snake position or who stands curled into a C-shape in close range to you. You can straighten her out (and knock her back) with a swift uppercut to the chin and then finish her off with a left hook. A person with a good right uppercut can make money boxing.

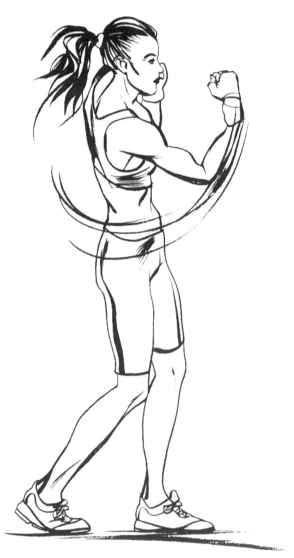

1. Start in snake position. Drop your right shoulder slightly and drop your right fist slightly, rotating it so your knuckles are facing up, toward the ceiling.
2. Push off the ball of your back foot pivoting your right hip forward, and follow through with your right fist, driving your knuckles in an upward motion into your opponent's chin.

**FOCUS**

Try to end the fight with this punch. If your opponent tilts forward—she's getting lazy in her body setup—her chin is hanging out in the open waiting to receive your uppercut. Go for it. This is a power punch—you can end the fight with this punch.

**ALWAYS**

◆ Keep your right arm at a 90-degree angle throughout the blow.
◆ Move close enough to your target so you can make a solid connection with this punch.

**NEVER**

◆ Drop your left hand.
◆ Cock your right hand back before the punch, so your fist starts by your ribs. You'll get hit, plus you're telegraphing your own punch.

# The Left Uppercut

## GOAL

This is a variation of the right uppercut and equally delivers a blow that is the punishment for any boxer who leans forward in snake position or who stands curled into a C-shape in close range to you. You need to be equally skilled at both right and left uppercuts, so you can take advantage of your best shot. You can straighten her out (and knock her back) with a swift uppercut to the chin and then finish her off with a right hook. A person with a good uppercut can become a contender. Basically, you are repeating the same motions as you would in performing a right uppercut, only you now switch sides.

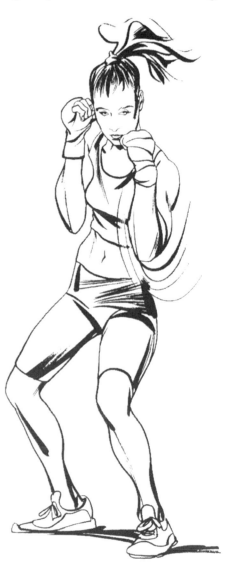

1. Start in snake position. Drop your left shoulder and left fist slightly, rotating your wrist so your knuckles are facing up, toward the ceiling.
2. Push off the ball of your back foot, pivoting your left hip forward, and follow through with your left fist, driving your knuckles in an upward motion into your opponent's chin.

**FOCUS**

This punch is not as powerful as the right uppercut. To end the fight with this punch, it must be used in combination with the jab and the left hook. If your opponent tilts forward—she's getting lazy in her body setup—her chin is hanging out in the open waiting to receive your uppercut. Go for it.

**ALWAYS**

◆ Keep your left arm at a 90-degree angle throughout the blow.
◆ Move close enough to your target so you can make a solid connection with this punch.

**NEVER**

◆ Drop your right hand.
◆ Cock your left hand back before the punch, so your fist starts by your ribs. You'll get hit, plus you're telegraphing your own punch

# ★ READ A PUNCH ★
## DON'T TELEGRAPH YOUR OWN

The smartest boxers are the ones who know what their opponent's next move is, but never let their opponents figure out theirs. That means you need to know how to read your opponent's punch and never telegraph your own. It takes a lot of practice to learn to read punches, pick up on your opponent's favorite combinations, think fast enough to defend yourself properly, and keep your punches hidden. Shadowboxing helps give your muscles the memory of throwing and defending against combinations in a split second, and doing it correctly helps you to stay in position to keep from giving away your next move. Try these tips to both read and avoid telegraphing punches.

### Reading Her Punches

1. Focus on the center of your opponent's body, from the neck to the upper chest, including the shoulder but not the arm. Her movements originate from this area, so keep your eye on it. If you look at her arm, fist, leg, or face, you're not concentrating.

2. Now think ahead. If you see the left shoulder extending, a jab is coming, so step to the left. If you see the right shoulder extending, a right hook or right cross is on its way to your face, so step to the right. Look for her elbow coming away from her ribcage and her forearm moving parallel to the floor—telltale signs of a hook—and squat down.

3. It's harder to read an uppercut because it's usually delivered by an opponent standing close to you.

4. Don't break your concentration. Remember, boxing is a mental sport, so you have to keep your focus laser-like. We see so many boxers stray for a split second—their eyes dart into the crowd, they

glance at the trainer, they look into their opponent's eyes—and that's when they get hit.

### Don't Telegraph Your Punches

1. Start in the snake position and return to it after you've thrown a punch. Snakes are sneaky; you don't know what they are going to do next so that should also be your goal.

2. Don't cock your fist back before you throw a punch. That's the biggest mistake new boxers make. It's also what guys do in a street fight, but you're in a controlled match—a sport—not a brawl. A good opponent will see that cocked fist coming a mile away.

3. Avoid looping your punches. Looping means, bringing your arm back and over. Move your arm and wrist straight through your punch without arching your arm. Think drill bit.

## Defensive Moves

Defense is the most crucial part of the game. If you can't defend yourself, you're going to end up on the wrong end of every punch. Get your feet right. Learn to move around quickly. In time, you'll learn to read punches, do what it takes to get out of the way of them, and counter with something fierce.

# The Duck

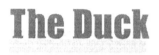

## GOAL

When your opponent delivers a left or right hook, you want to duck down below her fist so it swings above you. Spring back to snake position, ready to deliver your counterpunch. She'll be wide open.

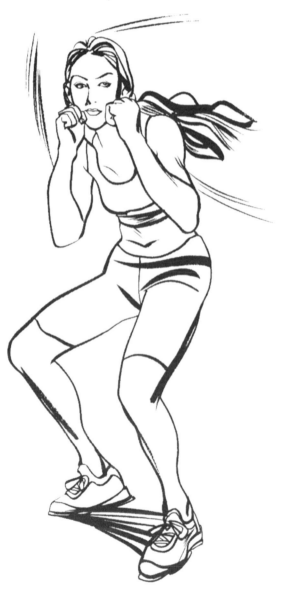

1. Start in snake position, legs straight, abs in, and eyes focused on your opponent.
2. Once her fist has swung above your head, return to snake position and prepare to return with a jab, cross, or hook.

**FOCUS** Never take your eyes off your opponent's face, even when you duck down, and be quick on your return. You want to spring back into the snake position, so you're ready to counter.

**ALWAYS**
◆ Keep your weight centered.
◆ Look directly at your opponent at all times.

**NEVER**
◆ Drop your head, or you'll be open for a punch.
◆ Lean forward or to either side as your squat, or you'll be knocked off balance.
◆ Allow your knees to extend past your toes, or you may injure your joints.

# The Slip

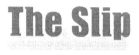

## GOAL

When your opponent delivers a jab or a right, twist your body to either side, so her fist completely misses you. As a result, you'll set yourself up for an easy counter-punch.

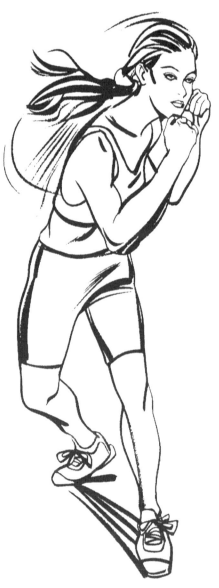

## STEP FOR SLIPPING A JAB (SLIP-RIGHT)

When your opponent's left fist comes at your chin, twist to your right, so your left shoulder turns toward your opponent's chest and her arm moves behind your back.

## STEP FOR SLIPPING A RIGHT (SLIP-LEFT)

When your opponent's right fist comes at your chin, twist to your left, so your right shoulder turns toward your opponent's, and her arm moves behind your back.

FOCUS    Concentrate on twisting from your core, so you don't have to pivot your back foot. Pivoting on a slip is old school, useful only if you were standing in the old-fashioned, upright position, which you should never do.

ALWAYS
◆ Turn into a punch, so it goes on your back, not your face or chest. You'll have a better shot at dodging it, and you'll be less likely to get knocked down.
◆ Keep your weight centered equally on both feet.
◆ Keep your fists at chin-level and your abs tight.

NEVER
◆ Turn away from a punch, or you'll open yourself up for another one.
◆ Lean back from a punch, or you'll get knocked off balance.

# The Elbow Block

## GOAL

When there's not enough time to get out of the way, you must prepare yourself to block a punch so it does the least amount of damage. The elbow block is what you should use any time your opponent aims for your body or sides, usually with a hook.

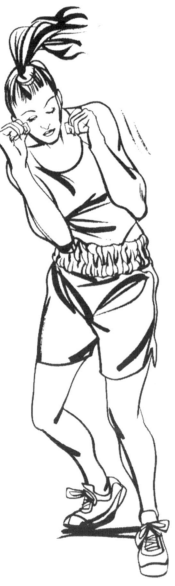

**STEPS**

1. Start in snake position, with your fists by your chin and your arms braced by your sides.
2. As your opponent's fist moves toward either of your sides, squat down, so the blow lands squarely on your elbow.

**FOCUS**

After you deflect the power of the punch, be prepared to counter immediately. An elbow block sets you up perfectly for an inside jab, using the same arm that's just been hit.

**ALWAYS**

◆ Bend from the knees, not the waist.
◆ Keep your torso upright.

**NEVER**

◆ Lean forward or to either side.
◆ Take your eyes off your opponent.
◆ Drop your fists.

**VARIATION**

If the punch is coming toward the center of your abs, rather than your ribs, quickly turn your body so the punch still lands on your elbow.

# Bobbing and Weaving

## GOAL

Bobbing and weaving mixes punch ducking with side-to-side movement. It throws your opponent off balance and puts you in a better position to counter.

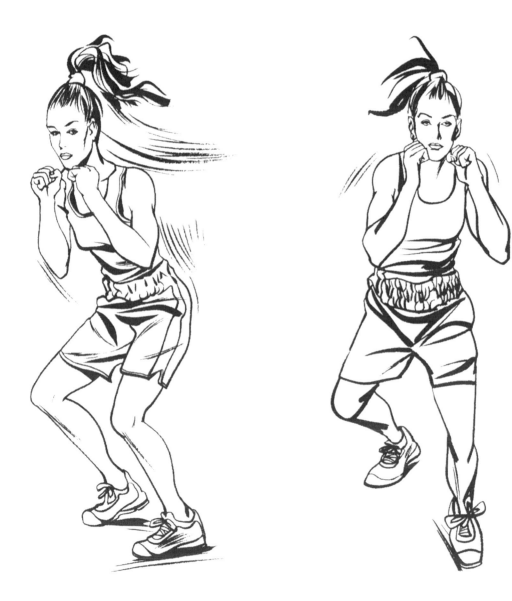

## EQUIPMENT REQUIRED

One 10- to 12-foot-long rope.

STEPS
1. Tie your rope between two points at shoulder height. You can use a couple of trees, hat racks, closet bars, or whatever you can find.
2. Stand in snake position just to the left of your rope.
3. Duck down (to avoid your opponent's punch, especially a right hook).
4. While still in the squat position, step to the right with your right foot, so your body moves to the other side of the rope. (This is the weave.)
5. Pop, or bob, up into snake position.

## FOR MORE ADVANCED FIGHTERS

Advance or retreat to any point on the rope, and repeat the bob and weave, alternating sides. Vary your movement each time.

FOCUS

Think of this maneuver as a setup for your offense because you're setting yourself up for your next move, not just getting out of the way of your opponent's fist. You should know what punch you're going to throw before you even rise from your squat position.

ALWAYS

◆ Keep your torso vertical. It's hard not to lean forward, but if you do, you'll be an easy target for your opponent's uppercut, and that hurts.
◆ Keep your eyes on your opponent.

NEVER

◆ Drop your fists.
◆ Jump out of your squat position. You never want to have both feet off the floor at once.

## Slipping Combinations

Throwing and slipping combination punches will become an essential part of your shadowboxing training in the coming weeks. We'll explain how to defend yourself against each type of combination in the workouts ahead, but for now, here's just a quick note. When you slip combinations—say, a one-two punch, which is a left jab followed by a straight right—you simply use the same defenses you would for a single punch. You already know and have practiced slipping by a left jab by turning to the right and slipping a right cross by turning to the left. So, to defend yourself against a one-two punch, you just combine both defense tactics: a quick twist to the right and a quick twist to the left. If your opponent comes at you with a jab and a left hook, you use a slip (to avoid the jab) and then a duck (to avoid the hook).

# Final Thoughts from Your Trainer

Even though on TV boxing looks like it is about brute strength, being a successful fighter takes more than just toughness. It also takes form. There is an art to this, and you can't step into the ring without knowing the proper form to use. That's why even if we see some big, tough, powerful street fighter who looks like he could take on anyone, we would never put that guy into the ring at Gleason's. No matter how strong he (or she) is, that fighter would get hammered without first knowing the basics—stance, footwork, punches, and defense—and how to do them properly.

If you practice enough, it just becomes habit. You won't have to think about each move so hard. For now, we can't emphasize this enough. Take it slow. Master your form. Don't rush it. If you don't have your technique down, you're going to get knocked down fast. You must be willing to put in the time, practice and do the same moves over and over until your form is correct. If you're not going to do it right, you're just wasting your own time and you don't belong in the sport.

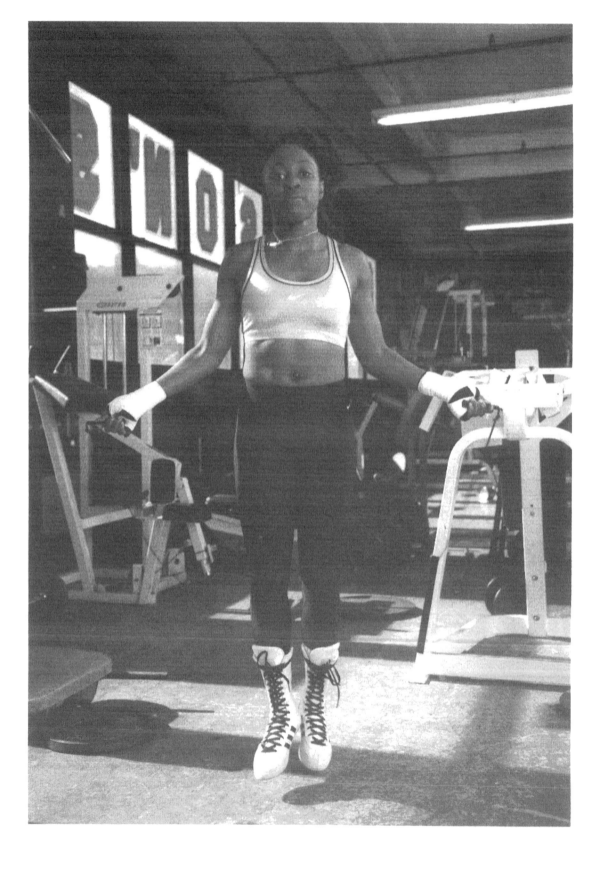

# 5
# Training Basics

**N**ow that you know the punches, you'll learn how fighters build power and stamina in preparation for entering the ring. In this chapter, we'll take you through each part of the workout preparation for actually beginning the program. You'll learn the most fundamental components of any boxing workout: strength training, shadowboxing, and jumping rope. Plus, we'll teach you how to stretch and build your cardiovascular fitness so that by the next chapter, you'll be ready to pull it all together and get started.

At Gleason's every fighter knows that being in top condition is critical to winning. Watch a boxing match, and it'll be clear: It's rarely the boxer with the hardest punches and the trickiest moves who'll win the fight. It's the one who's in the best shape, particularly near the end of the fight, the one who can go the distance is the one that becomes a champion. Champions are the ones who are hungry to be boxers. They give their all—and more. They dedicate themselves to their training and are driven, attentive, and alert at all times during their workouts. Once they step into the ring, they do just about everything right—not just because they are skilled. They throw punches correctly, defend themselves, keep moving, and remain focused because of their strength and stamina.

Please read this tutorial thoroughly before you get started with the workouts that are mapped out in the next chapters. Your workouts will go smoothly simply because you'll know what you're doing. There are three core components to each training session: jump rope, shadowboxing, and strength training—plus a warm-up and cooldown. During the first weeks, you'll work out for thirty minutes a session and then gradually build to forty-five minutes. Don't be fooled: It'll be tough at first because these workouts are vigorous. But you will see results: Your body will begin to look different; you'll be slimmer and leaner. You'll also be stronger and have more stamina. Mentally, you'll be more focused, self-confident, and happier. So let's get going.

## — COACH'S CORNER —

Boxing is a complete workout. If you train, and train hard, it will get you in the best shape of your life.

# Step 1: Get Loose:
## HOW TO STRETCH

You *must* stretch before you begin training. Your workouts will flow more easily if your muscles are warm and loose. More importantly, cold, tight, stiff muscles can lead to an injury. We've seen too many fighters hyped up on adrenaline who skip this step and end up sidelined. Even if you never plan to step into the ring, take the time to loosen up—starting at the top of your body and moving down. Be sure you spend at least five to seven minutes stretching, and longer if you have the time.

# ★ STRETCHING: THE RULES ★

Stretching is designed to prevent injuries, so stretch carefully to avoid causing one!

Get warm. It's always best to spend a few minutes running in place or doing some jumping jacks to warm up—and wake up—before you stretch. This will make your muscles warm and ready.

Go slow. Move into each position slowly. Moving too quickly or jerking will make your muscles tense up. So relax, and if you feel impatient, take a breath and think *slow motion*.

Don't bounce. Bouncing is natural to boxing, like when you're jumping rope or sparring, but it's all wrong for stretching. Instead, ease into your moves and hold your position for ten seconds or several breaths as you feel the tension drain from your muscles.

Pain isn't gain. Each stretch should feel relaxing, not painful. This isn't the time to push it and risk pulling a muscle. So, pay attention to your body and if something hurts, ease up.

Breathe deeply. Hold each position through at least two or three deep inhales and exhales. Deep breathing is a great way to release tension—in your muscles and your mind. Don't hold your breath; you want to be relaxed, not blue.

# ★ YOUR PRE-WORKOUT STRETCHING ROUTINE ★

We've offered you the following simple stretches. But you can also pick and choose others that you know and like. Just make sure your body parts feel relaxed and open.

## Neck

Keeping your shoulders relaxed, slowly lean your head toward your right shoulder. Use your right hand to very gently pull on the side of your head; stretch your left arm down your side. Hold through 2 deep breaths, then switch sides. Repeat.

## Shoulders

As you inhale deeply, raise the tops of your shoulders toward your ears. Exhale slowly and lower your shoulders. Repeat several times.

## Chest and Arms

Bring your arms behind you, and clasp your hands together. Keeping your shoulders relaxed and back straight, inhale deeply, raising your chest. You'll feel a pull across your chest. Exhale and relax. Repeat 3 or 4 times.

## Sides of the Body and Hips

Clasp your hands over your head loosely and bend to your right. Hold through 2 deep breaths. Keep your back straight and your knees bent slightly for balance. Slowly switch sides.

## Lower Back and Hamstrings

From a standing position with your feet about shoulder-width apart, bend forward from the hips. Keep your knees bent slightly, as you lower your arms toward the floor. Let your neck relax and feel a mild stretch in your lower back and the backs of your legs. Don't bounce. Take a couple of deep breaths, and then very slowly straighten to standing position. Keep your knees bent slightly; don't lock them. Repeat several times.

### Thighs and Knees

While standing, hold the top of your right foot with your left hand and gently pull your heel toward your butt. If you have trouble balancing, concentrate on a spot in front of you, or place your right hand against a wall. Or you can try this lying on your stomach. Take a couple of deep breaths, then switch legs. Repeat.

### Groin

Sitting down, get into a "butterfly" position by placing the soles of your feel together and holding your toes. Gently bend your back forward until you feel a mild stretch in your groin. Take several deep breaths and increase the stretch slightly. Don't bounce your legs.

### Calves

Standing about two feet from a wall, lean forward placing your hands on the wall. Bend your arms slightly and feel a gentle stretch in the muscles of both your calves. Tighten your abdominal muscles to avoid arching your back. Breathe deeply and increase the stretch by taking a step back from the wall or bending your arms more.

# Step 2: Jump on It

## JUMPING ROPE

First and foremost jumping rope builds cardiovascular endurance and gives boxers the stamina they need to last round after round. It also helps improve footwork, coordination, and balance. Muhammad Ali said that he loved skipping rope as part of his training. It helped perfect what he called his "prancing and dancing" in the ring.

Jumping rope isn't that tough, which is why kids love it so much. It's best to start out slow and steady, so you don't get tripped up—especially if you haven't jumped rope since your elementary school days. However, since our workout calls for quite a bit of jumping rope, building to twelve-minute sessions, you'll need to mix it by learning some footwork and arm moves. Before trying any tricks, keep these guidelines in mind:

◆ Keep it simple, relax, and find your rhythm.

◆ Jump with both feet and land on the balls of your feet.

◆ Lift your feet off the floor just high enough for the rope to pass quickly. Avoid jumping too high or landing too hard.

◆ Wear sneakers with plenty of padding to absorb the shock of your body weight. (Light-weight cross trainers or running shoes are best.) Always wear socks to prevent blisters.

◆ Bend your knees slightly, rather than locking them. This will help absorb the force of your body weight.

◆ Keep your shoulders relaxed and your hands at your sides and turn with your wrists—not with your arms.

◆ Be patient. Start out slowly, and then increase your speed once you become more comfortable.

## ★ THE RIGHT ROPE ★

There are many different kinds of jump ropes. When choosing the right one for you, make sure the length is correct. Hold the rope and stand with your feet on the middle. If the length is just right, the handles should just reach your armpits. The handles should be thick and comfortable.

Once you've gotten the hang of jumping, try running in place while turning the rope for variety and an additional challenge. Turn the rope and step over it with one foot. On the next turn, step over the rope with the other foot. You should feel like you're jogging in place while jumping rope.

## — COACH'S CORNER —

Why do you jump rope? That's just what boxers do.

Footwork, not punching, is the foundation of your boxing practice. Jumping rope improves footwork and balance. Skipping from foot to foot involved in jumping rope is great practice for shifting your weight into your punches.

"I used to hate jumping rope and not be able to do it. But after three months of getting laughed at, I now can jump for twenty minutes at a time!" —Alexis, age 23

# ★ HOW DO I KNOW HOW FAST TO GO? ★

It's important to gauge how hard your body is working, based on how you feel, not how you think you're supposed to feel. (For some people, walking up one flight of stairs is all it takes to get short of breath. For others, it'll take running up ten flights to get that same response.) That's why, when it comes to your rope skipping, we're not going to tell you how fast to turn the rope or how many jumps to squeeze in per minute. Instead, pace yourself based on your perceived level of exertion, using this one-to-ten scale:

## 1–2 Just Barely Moving

You're moving, but you're certainly not putting yourself out at all. Think window shopping or strolling through the park.

## 3–4 Easy

This is your brisk, warm-up pace. Your blood is pumping, and your muscles warm, but you're still breathing at or close to normal.

## 5–6 Moderate

Now, you're starting to work hard. You should feel your heart pounding and sweat forming on your forehead. You should also be breathing faster than normal, but not so hard that you can't hold a conversation without gasping for air between sentences.

## 7–8 Intense

You can feel your heart beating. You're breathing so heavily that you can't talk without pausing for air between phrases. In the ring, this is how you'll feel when you're going all out during the last thirty seconds of the last round.

## 9–10 All Out

You are performing at your body's maximum capacity, which you can only sustain for a very, very short period of time. (If ever you're working this hard, there is probably a hungry bear running toward you.)

For our program, you'll start out jumping at an easy pace, then move to a moderate level followed by an intense level. Because it's difficult to go 'all out' for very long, that level is too intense for our program. And if you're barely moving, you'll need to push harder to reap the full benefit of our program—which is short but intense.

# Step 3:
## SHADOWBOXING

You learned the moves in the previous chapter, and you'll put them into practice when you shadowbox. Shadowboxing builds both strength and stamina, and boxers use it to sharpen their skills and master their technique and form. It may feel awkward at first, but this is the best way to learn how to box. The more you practice, the more comfortable and natural you'll feel. It's just like being in a real fight with an imaginary opponent and is so second nature, that for boxers it's like walking. It's great to be your own opponent—and your own trainer—by boxing in front of a mirror. That way you can check your own form and technique and make sure that you're doing everything correctly, especially as you move from simple punches to more complicated combinations.

Here's some advice from Gleason's boxers on shadowboxing.

"Shadowboxing was very difficult for me, until I started thinking of it like a dance. Recently I went to a party for an old ballet teacher of mine, who is now eighty-nine. His daughter mentioned to me that he had studied boxing before he started ballet. When I put the connection between boxing and ballet in my head, shadowboxing got easier for me."
—Laila Ferioli, age 44

"I love shadowboxing. It's great for balance and for coordination."
—Jill Emery, age 35

"I have a dance background, so I learned to use movement to my advantage. It's an important part of my style."

—Three-time World Champion Alicia Ashley, age 38,

# Step 4: Power Up
## BUILDING YOUR STRENGTH

Fighters have long, lean muscles, and that's what you'll build with the strength moves in our workout. For boxers, being strong puts power behind the punch. In your everyday life, it means being able to walk up the stairs carrying three bags of groceries, preventing injuries of all kinds, speeding up your metabolism (muscle burns calories even when you're sitting still), and building healthy bones. Best of all, you'll look better—sleeker, slimmer, and more sculpted—and feel healthier and more confident.

There are lots of fancy "power moves," but our strength exercises are simple, low-tech, old school favorites. Sit-ups, push-ups, and other kinds of familiar, tested strength-training exercises are what we do, so we stand by them and stick to them. There is no point in changing the exercises that have worked for us for so long. Everybody that walks through the door at Gleason's does this workout. If you want to learn lots of new and fancy moves, put on some spandex and join a health club. But if you want to get strong and train as a fighter, then use what really leads to success.

The exercises we recommend in this book focus on your arms, chest, back, abdominals, and legs. You don't need any equipment except a mat for floor exercises and your own body. You won't bulk up too much by following the moves included in this chapter because they're designed to increase strength and agility, rather than create mass. Be careful not to hold your breath while you do these exercises. Breathing deeply will make performing these exercises easier. Let's get started.

— COACH'S CORNER —

Strength training is like vitamins for your muscles.

# Alligator Push-up

This strengthens upper body, particularly arms and shoulders.

All boxers do push-ups. They strengthen your upper body and can make the difference between a strong fighter and a weak one. The speed and force behind a punch comes from your shoulders, and push-ups build strong shoulders. A fighter who drops her hands and gets hit in the face is weak because she hasn't done enough push-ups.

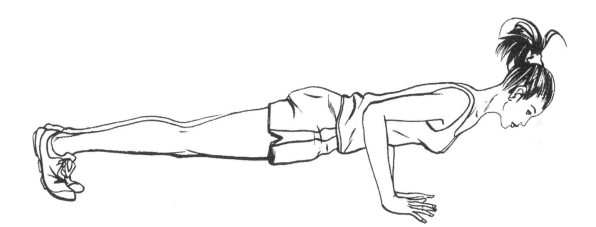

1. On your hands and knees, place your hands on the floor just above your waist, about 4 inches from your body on both sides. Moving your arms farther from the body makes the exercise easier, but we prefer arms closer.

2. Stretch your legs straight back, your toes curled under slightly, and your feet a few inches apart.

3. Keeping your body straight by using your abdominals, bend your arms and lower yourself to the ground, until you almost touch it. Your body should be straight, like a plank.

4. Push yourself back up again.

## FIT TIPS

◆ Be careful not to let your hips sag, your neck and head drop, or your back arch, or put your butt in the air. Think *straight back*, like a plank.

◆ Don't feel bad if you can't do a push-up right away, you can't do more than one or two, or your arms are shaking like crazy on the way up and down.

## EXERCISE ALTERNATIVE

If you don't have the upper-body strength to do push-ups, don't feel bad. It's better to start out slowly with a slightly easier exercise than to do the exercise incorrectly. So if you're having trouble, try these alternatives that will ease you into push-ups until you're strong enough to do the real thing.

## Modified Push-ups

Back in the day, these were known as girls' push-ups. You do these modified push-ups exactly as you would a regular push-up, but you support your weight by bending your knees.

1. On your hands and knees, place your hands on the floor just above your waist, about 4 inches from your body. Moving your arms farther from the body makes the exercise easier, but we prefer arms closer.
2. Rather than stretching your legs back, drop your knees to the floor. Your weight should be supported by your bent knees, rather than your toes.
3. Keeping the rest of your body straight by tightening your abdominals, bend your arms and lower yourself to the ground, until you almost touch it.
4. Push yourself back up again.

## Wall Push-ups

This is another, easier alternative: the wall push-up.

1. Lean on a wall with your hands shoulder-distance apart.
2. Bend your arms so that your nose almost touches the wall. As you're doing the exercise, remember to pull in your abdominal muscles.
3. Straighten your arms and repeat.

# Bicycle

This exercise strengthens your abs and firms up your leg muscles.

Lower body strength is a key component of boxing. If you can't move your feet quickly in the ring, you'll be a slow, easy target. And leg strength puts power behind the jab—boxing's most important punch.

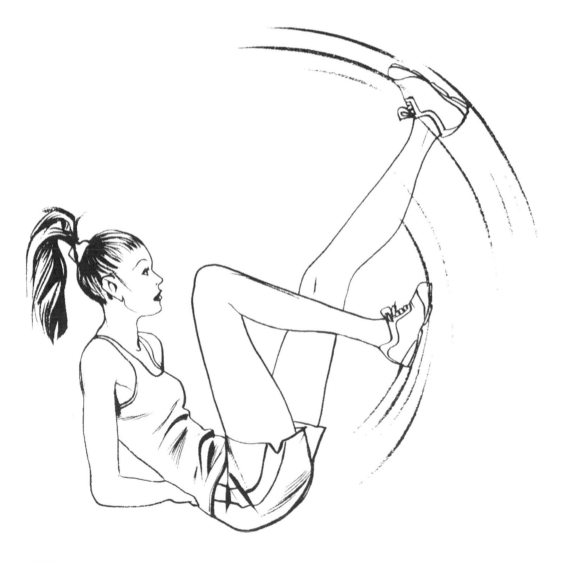

1. Lie face up with your lower back pressed to the floor and shoulders lifted very slightly—about an inch—off the ground.
2. Support your body weight with your elbows on the floor and your hands on your lower back just above your tailbone.
3. Raise your legs in the air, V-shaped. Bend one knee, then straighten it toward the ceiling without locking it.
4. Alternate your legs as if riding a bike.

## FIT TIPS

◆ Don't hold your breath while you're doing this exercise. Pretend like you're pedaling and breathe deeply.
◆ Be careful not to punch your legs in the air. The motion should be smooth.

## EXERCISE ALTERNATIVE

Try this for variety.

1. Lie face up with your lower back pressed to the floor.
2. Place your hands behind your head. Cradle your head in your hands, with your elbows out.
3. Bend your right knee, pulling it toward your chest (rather than up in the air) while touching the knee with the opposite elbow.
4. Continue this slow pedalling motion by touching your opposite elbow to your opposite knee, alternating each side.
5. Keep your abs pulled in and breathe continuously. Do 25 times on each side.

# The Bow

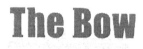

This yoga-inspired exercise strengthens and stretches your abdomen, your back, the fronts of your shoulders, and the fronts of your hips and thighs. It's isometric; in other words, you build strength by holding the position in place, rather than by moving. This will help you maintain the snake position, the key stance in boxing.

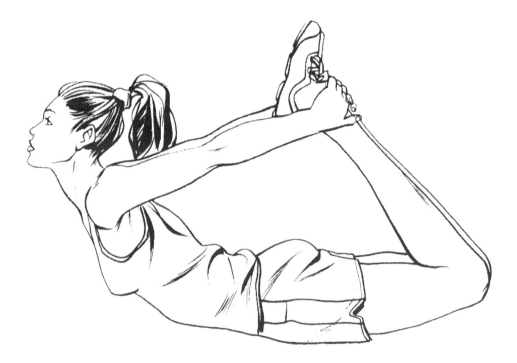

1. Lie on your stomach, bend your knees, and reach to your sides. Then reach backward and grab your ankles or shins.
2. Contract the muscles between your shoulder blades as well as your buttocks.
3. Use your arms to help hold you in position.

## FIT TIPS

◆ Keep your legs slightly apart if your back is not so flexible. Otherwise, keep the legs together.
◆ Make sure to start the movement with the contraction of muscles at the back of your body and not by pulling on your legs with your arms.
◆ Don't hold your breath.

## EXERCISE ALTERNATIVE

Mix it up with back extensions.

1. Lie face down with your hands either behind your back or lightly cradling your head.
2. Lift your upper body off the ground a few inches, keeping your head and neck in alignment.
3. For an extra challenge, lift your feet off the ground, keeping legs straight (knees don't have to be together). Hold for 2–4 counts and lower.

# Chest Push-up

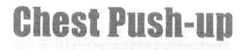

This gentle exercise strengthens not only your arms, but also your lower back. A strong core, including your lower back, will keep you steady on your feet and help you absorb punches to the body.

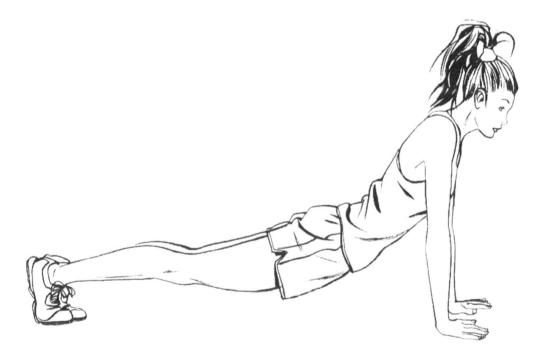

1. Lie on the floor with your abdomen pressed flat to the floor.
2. Place your hands flat on the floor, beneath your shoulders and shoulder-width apart. Your elbows should be at your sides.
3. Push your chest up with your arms, keeping them slightly bent, and hold this position for 10 seconds. Then lower yourself back to the floor.

## FIT TIPS

◆ Go slowly, taking deep breaths.
◆ Keep your abdomen tight to avoid back strain.

## EXERCISE ALTERNATIVE

Try the back extension.

1. Lie on your stomach. Place your arms at your sides so that your hands are by your hips.
2. Raise your head and shoulders off the mat as high as comfortably possible. Hold for 10 seconds.
3. Lower the head and shoulders. Do not tense your shoulder muscles.

# Crunch

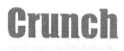

Crunches strengthen your abdominals. In boxing, you need strong abs so that you can take a body shot. If your middle is soft, it's going to hurt when you get hit there. There are lots of ways to do a crunch. This is the one we prefer at Gleason's.

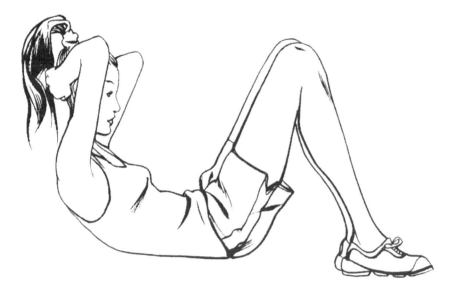

1. On the floor, lie on your back with your knees bent and hands behind your head.
2. Pull your belly button toward your spine by contracting your abs, while raising your head, neck, and shoulders about 2 or 3 inches off the floor, keeping your lower back flat to the floor.
3. Hold that position for a few minutes, while continuing to breathe.
4. Lower yourself slowly back to the floor.

## FIT TIPS

◆ Keep your neck straight—in line with your shoulders and upper back—to avoid straining yourself.
◆ Make sure your lower back stays on the floor during the entire exercise.

## EXERCISE ALTERNATIVE

For a change, try a crunch with a twist.

1. On the floor, lie on your back with your knees bent and hands behind your head.
2. Contract your abs, while raising your head, neck, and shoulders about 2 or 3 inches off the floor.
3. As you roll up, add a twist by reaching your right elbow to your left knee. Keep your lower back flat to the floor.
4. Hold that position for a few minutes, while continuing to breathe.
5. Lower yourself slowly back to the floor. Repeat using your opposite elbow and knee. Do 30 times.

# Flutter Kicks

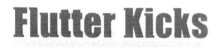

This exercise builds your abdominals so that you can receive a body shot without getting hurt and also strengthens your hip muscles, which will increase your power when you step and punch.

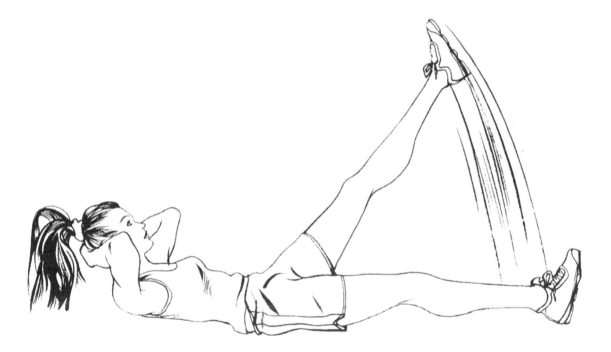

1. Lie face up with your lower back pressed firmly to the floor, with your hands behind your head.
2. Lift your head and legs a few inches from the floor.
3. Tighten the abdominals and then alternate your legs up and down—not too fast—in a kicking motion without letting them touch the floor.

## FIT TIPS

◆ Be careful not to tense your neck or strain your lower back.

◆ As an alternative, rather than kicking your legs up and down, cross them sideways.

◆ At the end of your workout, hold your feet together 6 inches from the floor for 30 seconds. As your stamina improves, you can increase the time to 1 minute. For an advanced move, try holding your arms at either side 6 inches off the ground and imitate the movement of your legs.

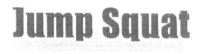

# Jump Squat

This is a plyometric exercise, which builds explosive power. It strengthens the thighs, calves, and gluts (in the buttocks), which will help keep you steady on your feet when you receive a blow and also build your lower body for better, faster footwork.

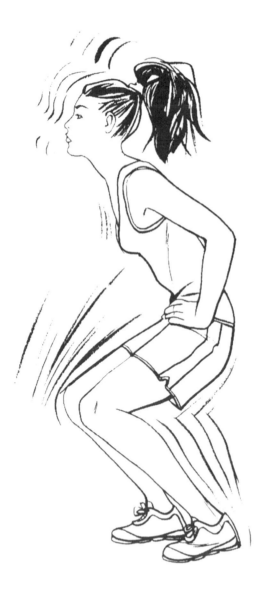

1. Stand with your hands on your hips, your head up, your back straight, and your feet about shoulder-width apart.
2. Bend your knees and squat until your thighs are about parallel to the floor.
3. Jump as high as you can straight up; think of your thighs as springs.
4. When you land on the floor, pause briefly and then repeat.

## FIT TIPS

◆ Be careful to land on the balls of your feet to absorb the shock from the weight of your body.

◆ Wear shoes and socks when you do this exercise.

## EXERCISE ALTERNATIVE

If you've had knee problems in the past, or for an alternative method that strengthens the same muscles, try the standing squat.

1. Stand with your hands on your hips, while keeping your back straight.
2. Bend your knees and squat until your thighs are about parallel to the floor.
3. Hold the position and then straighten up.

# Leg Raises

This exercise also strengthens the abdominals, again, which is key to withstanding a body shot.

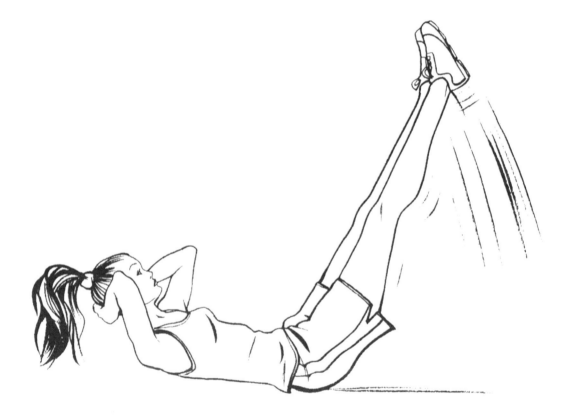

1. Lie face up with your back pressed firmly on the floor and your hands behind your head.
2. Raise your legs, with your knees bent slightly, about a foot off the floor and then hold them there.
3. Using just your lower abdominals, tilt your hips and raise your legs higher so that they are not quite at a 90-degree angle with the floor.
4. Hold the position for a few seconds, while continuing to breathe.
5. Lower your legs to about a foot off the floor and then hold the position again, before raising them. Do 20 straight reps.

## FIT TIPS

◆ Be careful not to strain your neck.
◆ If you feel a strain in your back, place the hands under your lower back, rather than behind the head.

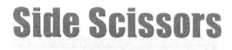

This exercise strengthens your hip, thigh, and groin muscles, which provides for added stability and steady movement in the ring. It also firms your sides, which enables you to absorb blows to the body.

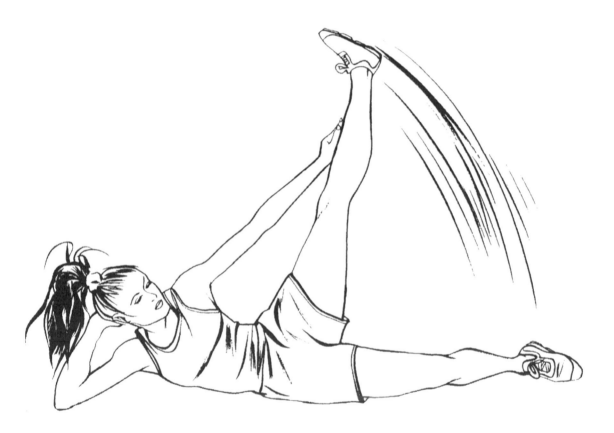

1. Lie on your right side with your right leg bent slightly.
2. Rest the side of your head in your right hand, with your right elbow on the floor.
3. Slowly lift your left leg 8–10 inches, then lower it slowly. Repeat several times. Turn over and repeat on your left side, raising your right leg.

## FIT TIPS

◆ Move through this exercise slowly, which is harder than racing through it quickly.

◆ Keep your balance by aligning your hips and shoulder.

◆ Occasionally, hold your foot in one position and twist it in either direction so that you hit different muscle groups. For an advanced move, kick your leg backward instead of vertically—this will work your glute muscles. To steady yourself during the movement, place your lower arm above your head and your upper arm in front of your body.

# Superman

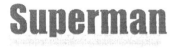

This strengthens your lower back, so you can maintain stability during punches and movement, and it works the chest and shoulders to put power behind your punches.

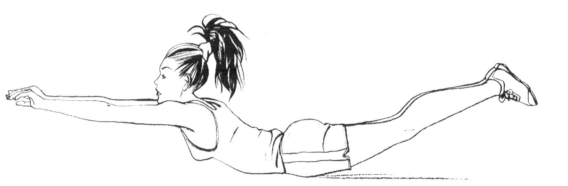

1. Lie face down on the floor, with your forehead and toes on the floor, and your arms extended out in front of your head.
2. Raise your head, chest, arms, and legs off the floor as high as you can without straining yourself—about 3 inches.
3. Hold that position for 3 seconds, then lower your chest, head, arms, legs, and toes to the floor. Repeat.

## FIT TIPS

◆ Strain isn't gain. If you feel a pain in your neck or back, lower your body slightly.

◆ Keep your head facing straight ahead, rather than looking up or down.

## EXERCISE ALTERNATIVE

Lift one leg and arm at a time if raising both is too difficult.

1. Lie face down on the floor, your forehead and toes touching the floor, and your arms extended out in front of your head.
2. Raise your head, chest, right arm, and left leg off the floor as high as you can without straining yourself—about 3 inches.
3. Hold that position for 3 seconds, then return chest, head, arms, legs, and toes to the floor. Repeat, switching to your left arm and right leg.

# Triangle Push-up

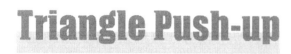

This is another push-up that's great for strengthening your upper body. It will help put more force behind your punches.

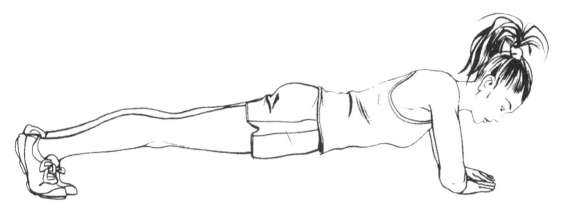

1. On your hands and knees, place your hands on the floor in front of your forehead, with your fingers and thumbs touching to form a triangle.
2. Stretch your legs straight back, with your toes curled under slightly and feet a few inches apart.
3. Keeping your body straight by using your abdominals, bend your arms and lower yourself to the ground, until you almost touch it. Your body should be straight, like a plank, with your face looking at the triangle your hands have formed.
4. Push yourself back up again. Do 15 straight reps.

## FIT TIPS

◆ Be careful not to let your hips sag, your neck and head drop, or your back arch, or put your butt in the air. Think *straight back,* like a plank.

◆ Don't feel bad if you can't do a push-up right away, you can't do more than one or two, or your arms are shaking like crazy on the way up and down.

## EXERCISE ALTERNATIVE

You can do the same exercise leaning against a wall.

### Wall Triangle Push-Ups

1. Lean your hands on a wall. Your fingers and thumbs should be touching to form a triangle.
2. Bend your arms so that your nose almost touches your fingers. As you're doing the exercise, remember to pull in your abdominal muscles.
3. Straighten arms and repeat.

# Walking Lunges

This strengthens the hips, thighs, and legs, and helps you focus on the proper boxing stance.

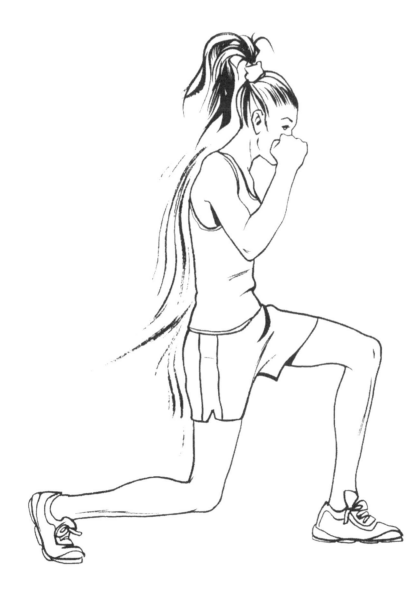

1. Start in the snake position by standing with your feet shoulder-width apart and your weight centered.

2. Raise both fists to chin level, palms facing inward with your elbows tight to your sides to protect your ribs.

3. Tuck your chin toward your chest and direct your gaze forward at your target, like you're looking through your eyebrows.

4. Keeping your upper body in the snake stance, start at one end of the room and take a long stride forward with the right leg.

5. Bend down so the forward knee is directly over the toes at a 90-degree angle.

6. Raise up and keep repeating while alternating with the other leg until you cross the room.

## FIT TIPS

◆ Keep your eyes focused on a point in the front of the room, so you don't lose your balance.

◆ Stay in the snake position. This is great practice for shadowboxing.

◆ Don't walk too fast. Pay attention to your form, not your speed.

# Parting Shots

The vast majority of fights don't end in a knockout. Most fighters will have to go the distance, which requires strength and stamina. You can see the signs of an out-of-shape fighter right away. Her arms will be dropped to her sides because she doesn't have the strength to hold them up and protect herself. She won't be dancing, but more like staggering, like she's had too much to drink. She'll look slow and miss punches, leaving herself open. And she'll be panting and sucking air, with her mind unfocused. We never put a fighter into the ring if she's weak or lacks cardiovascular fitness. It's not fair, and it's not safe. That's why we demand that all of our fighters train and train hard. A good fighter is self-motivated and driven toward her goal. She wants to have the feeling of power and freedom that comes with strength and stamina. That's what we want you to feel—invincible. You can only feel this way by sticking to the program and getting into shape.

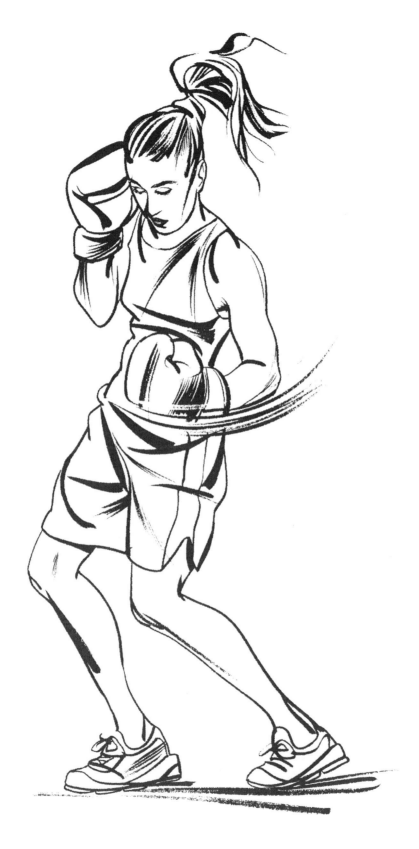

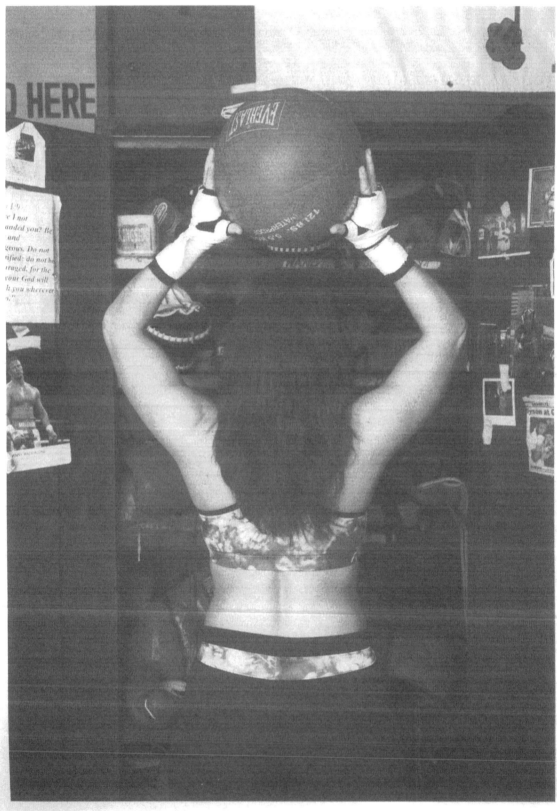

# 6
# Week One:
## Build Your Foundation

Now that you are beginning to master your strength and boxing moves, it's time to put them in motion. The real work behind your four-week better body makeover begins right here.

## How It Works

In the following pages, you'll find three, thirty-minute workouts for Week One. Each training session, this week and every week, comes in three easy-to-follow sections: jumping rope, shadowboxing, and strength training. You can do the workouts on consecutive days or take a day or two of rest in between. Just do them in order because each workout builds on the previous one.

# Find Your Focus

As you learned in chapter 2, mastering the mental part of boxing is half the fight. That's why it's important to come to each workout with a specific focus. If you know precisely what you want to accomplish during your session, you'll be more likely to go harder (and burn more calories), push through when you're tired, and sharpen specific fighting skills. If you just plan on going through the motions, don't bother doing the workout at all. You're just wasting your own time. You won't burn many calories. You won't build lean muscles. You certainly won't become a boxer. If you plan on giving it your all and you really pay attention to your form and movement, you'll learn plenty and burn many calories this week.

Each week, we'll give you two things to focus on: one fighting goal and one fitness goal. Read them over before each workout. Here are this week's objectives.

## Your Fighting Focus: Learn the Dance

This week's emphasis is squarely on defense and dancing, which means moving around the ring swiftly and lightly. Movement is the foundation of a good boxer, so it's important to do it the right way. Many fighters think that if they have a good jab or a good left hook, they're golden, but that's one of the biggest misconceptions in boxing. You need to be able to *create* the time and space to attack. If you can't avoid your opponent's punches, it doesn't matter how good, fast, or powerful yours are. You'll never get a chance to throw them. So, let's learn to dance.

## Your Fitness Focus: Find Your Footing

Baby steps. That's the key to getting fit and staying fit. If you start too hard or expect too much of yourself right away, you're going to get discouraged and quit. There's no room for quitters in the boxing ring! So this week's cardio—six minutes of jumping rope each day, plus two rounds of shadowboxing—is designed to build up slowly your endurance, your foot turnover, and your ego.

Everybody thinks jumping rope is easy. They think that if an eight-year-old girl can do it, they sure as hell can do it. Well, it's not quite *that* easy. It takes patience, coordination, agility, a strong sense of timing, and stamina—all boxing essentials.

So this week, just get used to handling a rope. If you get tripped up, take a deep breath and start again. Don't try to kill yourself with speed; it's more important to do it consistently. Go slow enough that you're always moving and keeping your heart rate up.

## ★ BEFORE YOU GET STARTED ★

### Four Points to Understand Before You Begin This Training Program

1. Stretch before and cool down after every workout. Both may be easy to do, but they are both equally as important to your health, fitness, and fighting ability as every other part of this workout. They'll keep your muscles loose and help prevent injury. Stretch from your head to your toes with the stretching program presented in chapter 5.

2. Work the bell. All of the cardio portions of these workouts come in three-minute intervals because every round in boxing is three minutes long. The boxer's body has muscle memory; it learns what three minutes feel like, and it eventually develops the ability to go harder for that short period of time, knowing it'll get a rest afterward. At Gleason's, we have boxing bells that go off every three minutes. At home, set an egg timer, your watch, or the timer on your stove—anything that can be easily set and you can see and hear will do.

3. Follow the Pyramid Principle. This is very important. Every workout builds on skills that you practiced previously. As you progress through this program, be sure to incorporate the moves that you worked on in each of

the previous workouts into your new shadowboxing routines. For example, in your first workout this week, you'll just concentrate on your footwork. In your second workout, you'll work on ducking and slipping. It's up to you to keep practicing the footwork during your ducking and slipping drills. By the end of this four-week program, you should be putting together everything you learned from the first workout of the first week through the last workout of the fourth week.

## ★ DRINK UP! ★

The average woman sweats out about one to two liters of water every hour during intensive cardio workouts. That means you need to drink five to eight ounces of water every fifteen minutes to stay properly hydrated. Take a few sips during every one-minute rest period.

## — COACH'S CORNER —

Be realistic about your goals. Do not overreach yourself. Do not use rubber or plastic suits to sweat excessively or to try to lose weight too quickly. It is dangerous; you risk dehydration and electrolyte imbalance. The weight will come off naturally with your training routine.

# The Workouts: Week One

## Day Two:
MASTER THE DANCE

## The Overview

Fast footwork—not punching—is the foundation of your boxing practice, and that's the skill you're going to work on today. During your shadowboxing rounds, you'll learn to run the cross and run the circle. These drills focus more on moving properly in the ring than hitting. Fitness-wise, this workout is the easiest one you'll do all month. And remember, even if you're not shedding buckets of sweat today—don't worry, that day will come—you're taking an extremely crucial step toward your fitness- and skill-level. Because of that, it'll be easy to just sail through the motions. Don't do it. Focus your mind before you start because boxing-wise, this is the most important workout you'll do. Today, you'll begin the process of learning what made Muhammad Ali so great.

## — COACH'S CORNER —

I like a boxer who's a little flashy in the feet because it frustrates the opponent. But you also have to be able to put together some punches, or that fancy footwork isn't worth a thing.

# ★ MASTERING YOUR MOVES ★

Footwork doesn't have to be fancy—though it can be. Here are some tips for better movement.

Some boxers like Ali and Sugar Ray Leonard are known for their footwork. Although a great boxer doesn't have to be a great "dancer," we like fighters who move with a little bit of style and finesse. But proper movement is more than just entertainment: You have to have good footwork to move in tight and deliver solid punches. Even more importantly, you need to be fast on your feet to defend yourself and avoid getting hit. The key is to *keep movement efficient,* so that you control the center of the ring. Make your opponent waste movements, and she'll get tired and lose the fight. Here's how.

- As you practice your footwork, move quickly and change your directions sharply. That's how real boxers throw off their opponents.
- Be sure to maintain the proper form through each move. That means focus on what all of the parts of your body are doing, not just your feet.
- Stay on the balls of your feet—not your toes and definitely not your heels.
- Be light, not flat-footed, by visualizing floating on your feet.

# What You're Going to Do Today:

## WEEK ONE, DAY ONE

Here's what you're going to do today. Everything you need to know is in the next couple of pages. Tape this rundown to your mirror before you start, so you don't have to glance at the book between rounds. We'll walk you through every step, but we can't do it for you. It's up to you to commit to the workout and do it the right way.

# The Workout:

## WEEK ONE, DAY ONE

| | | |
|---|---|---|
| 6 Minutes: | Jump Rope | *Steady@Level 3–4* |
| 1 Minute: | Rest | |
| 3 Minutes: | Shadowboxing | *Run the Cross* |
| 1 Minute: | Rest | |
| 3 Minutes: | Shadowboxing | *Run the Circle* |
| 1 Minute: | Rest | |
| 15 Minutes: | Strength Training | |
| | *Jump Squats:* | *3 sets of 8* |
| | *Alligator Push-ups:* | *3 sets of 5* |
| | *Side Scissors:* | *3 sets of 10* |
| | *Crunches:* | *3 sets of 10* |

# The Details

## 6 Minutes: Jump Rope

Jumping rope is still probably new to you, so don't worry too much about your speed. Don't try anything fancy and just get the hang of the movement. Shoot for a level 3 or 4 of exertion, which is an easy pace. You should be out of breath but not falling to the floor. If you trip (and you will), don't get frustrated; that's not going to get you anywhere. Every single person in Gleason's gym has tripped on a jump rope. Nobody cries or whines. Just pick up the rope, start over, and jump until your six minutes are up. It will get easier.

## 1 Minute: Rest

Between real rounds of boxing you sit in your corner and rest for one minute. That's what you're going to do here, too. Resting doesn't mean taking a nap. Keep your head in it by imagining yourself as a fighter and visualizing your success. Walk around. Shake out your arms and legs.

## 3 Minutes: Shadowboxing
## Drill: Run the Cross

Goal: This left-right-advance-retreat drill, designed to help you master your movement, will teach you to float around the ring with speed and agility.

Three minutes is going to feel like a long time when you're advancing, retreating, and moving side-to-side, but you've got to do it until it feels like second nature. If you don't learn to move about the ring properly, you'll have absolutely no chance in a fight.

### Steps

1. Start in snake position with your weight centered. Shuffle to the left by taking a small step with your left (front) foot, followed by your right (back) foot. Repeat 3 times.

2. Shuffle back to the right, stepping first with your right (back) foot and then your left (front) foot. Repeat 3 times, bringing you back to where you started.

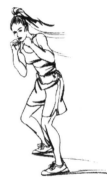

3. Advance toward your (real or imaginary) opponent by stepping forward first with your left (front) foot and quickly following with your right (back) foot. Repeat 3 times.

4. Retreat by stepping back first with your right (back) foot and then your left (front) foot. Repeat 3 times, until you return to your starting position.

5. Repeat the entire sequence 5 more times, and then switch the order. Move right, left, retreat, and advance. Repeat 5 times. Change order and repeat.

## 1 Minute: Rest

## 3 Minutes: Shadowboxing
## Drill: Run the Circle

Goal: To learn to move in a circle in the ring. Concentrate on switching directions quickly. Add feints—a quick shoulder dip to fake out your opponent—to bust up your predictability. The element of surprise is one of your best assets, so you never want to let your opponent know where you're going to go before you actually move.

## Steps

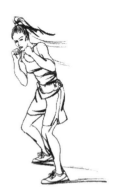

1. Recruit either a friend, who will stand still for you for 2 minutes, or a chair. Either will work just fine.

2. Assume the snake position and face your opponent (your pal or the chair).

3. Begin to circle, clockwise, by stepping to the left with your left (front) foot and following with your right (back) foot. Be careful not to cross your feet, which will put you off balance. The motion is more like a shuffle.

4. Continue slowly around your opponent until you're back to your starting position.

5. Switch directions, by stepping to the right with your right (back) foot, followed by your left (front) foot. Go around twice; switch direction and repeat; switch direction and repeat.

## 1 Minute: Rest

## 15 Minutes: Strength Training

In the cardio and shadowboxing parts of the workout, you'll mimic what happens in the ring with 3-minute intervals and 1-minute rest periods, so you know what a fight feels like. But boxers strength train on their own time. Building strong muscles has nothing to do with the clock; it's about pushing yourself to build strength on your own time. During strength training, rest 30 seconds between each set, and 1 minute between each exercise. This should challenge your muscles but also give them time to recover.

Concentrate on your form. With the exception of the jump squat, which requires explosive power, go through each step of every move slowly to get the maximum results.

### Jump Squats

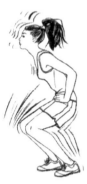

*Do 3 sets of 8.*

1. Stand with your hands on your hips, your head up, your back straight, and your feet about shoulder-width apart.

2. Bend knees and squat until your thighs are about parallel to the floor.

3. Jump as high as you can straight up; think of your thighs as springs.

4. When you land on the floor, pause briefly, and then repeat.

## Alligator Push-ups

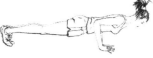

*Do 3 sets of 5. Do this exercise with knees bent instead of out straight if you need to.*

1. On your hands and knees, place your hands on the floor just above your waist, about 4 inches from both sides of your body. Moving your arms farther from the body makes the exercise easier, but we prefer arms closer.
2. Stretch your legs straight back, with your toes curled under slightly, and your feet a few inches apart.
3. Keeping your body straight by using your abdominals, bend your arms and lower yourself to the ground, until you almost touch it.
4. Push yourself back up again.

## Side Scissors

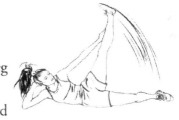

*Do 3 sets of 10.*

1. Lie on your right side with your right leg bent slightly.
2. Rest the side of your head in your right hand and elbow on the floor.
3. Slowly lift your left leg 8–10 inches then lower slowly. Repeat several times. Turn over and repeat on your left side, raising your right leg

## Crunches

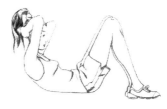

*Do 3 sets of 10.*

1. Lie on the floor on your back with your knees bent and your hands behind your head.
2. Pull your belly button toward your spine by contracting your abs, and then raise your head, neck, and shoulders about 2 or 3 inches off the floor. Keep your lower back flat to the floor.
3. Hold that position for a few minutes, while continuing to breathe.
4. Lower yourself slowly back to the floor.

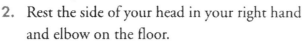

# Day Two:
SLIP PUNCHES

## The Overview

You'll add to your defensive repertoire today by learning to duck and slip punches. The squatting and twisting motions work your thighs and abs (especially your obliques) pretty hard, making this workout much more challenging than the previous one. (Don't be surprised if you feel a bit sore tomorrow or the next day.)

## What You're Going to Do Today:
WEEK ONE, DAY TWO

| | | |
|---|---|---|
| 6 Minutes: | Jump Rope | *Steady@Level 4–5* |
| 1 Minute: | Rest | |
| 3 Minutes: | Shadowboxing *Stationary Bobbing and Weaving* | |
| 1 Minute: | Rest | |
| 3 Minutes: | Shadowboxing | *Slip, Squat, Slip* |
| 1 Minute: | Rest | |
| 15 Minutes: | Strength Training *Bicycle: 3 sets of 40* *Bow: 1 set of 3, 10-second holds* *Triangle Push-Ups: 3 sets of 5* *Flutter Kicks: 3 sets of 12* | |

# The Details

## 6 Minutes: Jump Rope

Today, try stepping up your jump rope pace just a slight bit, moving from an exertion level of 3 or 4 to a level of 4 or 5. To make it a bit more challenging, either speed up the pace at which you swing the rope, or if you're tripping up a lot, speed your recovery. That is, start up again faster.

## 1 Minute: Rest

During the rest period you've got to prepare for the drill in your next 3-minute bout of shadowboxing during which you'll focus on bobbing and weaving. Find a short length of rope, clothesline, twine, or even ribbon (about 3 feet long) and tie it at shoulder height between two objects like a stair railing and a bookshelf, a coat rack and closet bars, or two trees if you're outside.

## 3 Minutes: Shadowboxing
## The Drill: Stationary Bobbing and Weaving

Goal: Mixing side-to-side movement with punch ducking.

Bobbing and weaving throws your opponent off balance and puts you in better position to counter. Remember that when you squat, don't do it like you're standing in molasses. Imagine a mean right hook coming at your head and—woosh!—drop down quickly. Side-step swiftly and pop up on the opposite side of the rope in snake position, ready to counter attack. Here's how to do it.

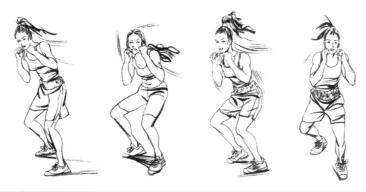

1. Stand in snake position just to the left of your rope.
2. Duck down (to avoid your opponent's punch, especially a right hook).
3. While still in the squat position, step to the right with your right foot, so your body moves to the other side of the rope. (This is the weave.)
4. Pop, or bob, up into snake position.

## 1 Minute: Rest

## 3 Minutes: Shadowboxing
## The Drill: Slip, Squat, Slip

Goal: Avoid your opponent's punches without getting too tired.
You slip jabs or rights and you duck hooks, and since all of those punches often come together, it's important to be able to defend yourself against the combinations. Again, eventually, you're going to add footwork to this drill, but for now, just practice your moves in one spot.

### Steps

1. Stand in snake position, preferably in front of a full-length mirror.
2. Slip to the right and return to snake position.
3. Squat and return to snake position. Remember to keep your torso vertical—don't bend over—fists up by your chin, and eyes on your imaginary opponent.
4. Slip to the left, squat, and return to snake position.
5. Do as many as you can for 3 minutes without losing your form. If you start bending forward or barely squatting, slow down and do it right.

## 1 Minute: Rest

## 15 Minutes: Strength Training

You never want to work the same muscles in the same way two days in a row, so you'll do four new strength moves today, which will work your body from different angles. Rest for 30 seconds between sets and 1 minute between moves.

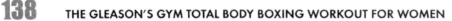

## Bicycle

*Do 3 sets of 40.*

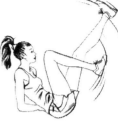

1. Lie face up with your lower back pressed to the floor and your shoulders lifted very slightly—about an inch—off the ground.
2. Support your body weight with your elbows on the floor and your hands on your lower back just above your tailbone.
3. Raise your legs in the air, V-shaped. Bend 1 knee, then straighten it toward the ceiling without locking it.
4. Alternate legs as if riding a bike.

## Bow

*Do 1 set of 3, holding the pose for 10 seconds and resting for 10 seconds between each rep.*

1. Lie on your stomach, bend your knees, and reach to your sides. Then reach backward and grab your ankles or shins.
2. Contract the muscles between your shoulder blades as well as your buttocks.
3. Use your arms to help hold you in position.

## Triangle Push-ups

*Do 3 sets of 5. Use your knees if need be.*

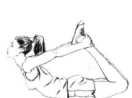

1. On your hands and knees, place your hands on the floor in front of your forehead, with your fingers and thumbs touching to form a triangle.
2. Stretch your legs straight back, with your toes curled under slightly and feet a few inches apart.
3. Keeping your body straight by using your abdominals, bend your arms and lower yourself to the ground, until you almost touch it. Your body should be straight, like a plank, with your face looking at the triangle your hands have formed.
4. Push yourself back up again.

## Flutter Kicks

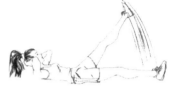

*Do 3 sets of 12.*

1. Lie face up on the floor with your lower back pressed firmly to the floor and your hands behind your head.
2. Lift your head and legs a few inches from the floor.
3. Tighten your abdominals and then alternate your legs up and down—not too fast—in a kicking motion without letting them touch the floor.

## ★ WATCH YOURSELF ★

When shadowboxing, always focus on your form by watching yourself closely in the mirror. Otherwise, you're going to start picking up bad habits. Here are the worst of the bad habits that we see over and over at the gym.

• Leaning forward or back: Keep your torso upright whenever you squat. Leaning forward or backward sets you up for getting knocked out. To move vertically, bend and straighten your knees.

• Dropping your hands: Between punches, stay in the snake position with your hands near your chin. Otherwise, you leave your face open to be hit.

• Closing your eyes: Always keep your eyes open when you punch even if you're only aiming at your reflection in the mirror.

• Crossing your feet: If you cross your feet when moving in the ring, you'll trip. Shuffle from side to side instead.

• Lifting your head when you throw a punch: Don't raise your head when you throw a punch. You'll throw yourself off balance, and your eyes will be off your opponent.

# Day Three:
## MIX UP YOUR DEFENSE

# The Overview

During the first workout of this week, you learned how to move around the ring. In the second workout, you practiced a few basic defensive moves. Today, you're going to work on putting both of those skills together. It's important that the movements you practice today become automatic for you. You want to do them so many times that you can box in your sleep without thinking *How do I punch? How do I move? What should I do next?* That's what turns a good fighter into a champion. During this session, you'll work your abs and legs, and you'll get your heart rate up and burn lots of calories.

# What You're Going to Do Today:
## WEEK ONE, DAY THREE

| 6 Minutes: | Jump Rope | *Steady@Level 5* |
|---|---|---|
| 1 Minute: | Rest | |
| 3 Minutes: | Shadowboxing | *Bob, Weave, and Move* |
| 1 Minute: | Rest | |
| 3 Minutes: | Shadowboxing | *Move and Slip, Squat, Slip* |
| 1 Minute: | Rest | |
| 15 Minutes: | Strength Training | |
| | *Walking Lunges: 3 sets of 10* | |
| | *Chest Push-ups: 3 sets of 5* | |
| | *Leg Raises: 3 sets of 10* | |
| | *Supermans: 1 set of 3* | |

# The Details

## 6 Minutes: Jump Rope

You should be getting a little better at the jump rope by now. So in this session, concentrate on tripping less and keeping an even-keeled pace (about a level 5) throughout the 6 minutes. You want to feel warm and loose, not exhausted, by the end of this round.

## 1 Minute: Rest

You've got another chore during this rest to get ready for bobbing and weaving. String up the rope again. Last time you used 3 feet of rope, but this time you'll need a longer piece—about 10 to 15 feet of it at shoulder height, so you can adequately move around.

## 3 Minutes: Shadowboxing
## The Drill: Bob, Weave, and Move

For the next round, mix up your bobbing and weaving with different lengths of advancing and retreating. Here's how to do it.

1.  Stand in snake position just to the left of your rope.
2.  Duck down (to avoid your opponent's punch, especially a right hook).
3.  While still in the squat position, step to the right with your right foot, so your body moves to the other side of the rope. (This is the weave.)

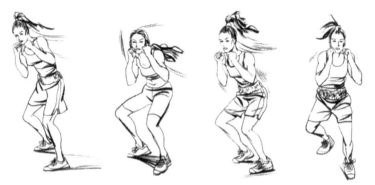

4.  Pop, or bob, up into snake position.

5. Move forward along the entire length of your rope, and then bob and weave to the other side.

6. Keep moving forward and backward along the rope, bobbing and weaving. You can choose how many steps you take, but try to do at least 1 or 2 steps forward or backward before bobbing and weaving. Or, advance, then retreat, then advance again, and bob and weave.

7. When you feel comfortable moving forward and backward, try circling out from the rope, and bob and weave when you get to it.

Try this combination:
1. Move halfway up the rope; bob and weave.
2. Continue moving forward, circle out, then bob and weave at the end of the rope.
3. Move backward half way, bob and weave, circle out on the other side of the rope and then bob and weave at the end.

Remember: Mixing up your movements like this keeps your opponent from knowing your next move. You know what that means: It keeps her fist off your face.

## 1 Minute: Rest

## 3 Minutes: Shadowboxing
## The Drill: Running the Cross, Slipping, and Squatting

Now that you've got the basic defensive maneuvers down—the slip and the squat—it's up to you to incorporate movement with them. Run the cross or the circle and add slip, squat, slip bursts at any point throughout the drill. If you're having trouble visualizing what you want to do at first, try first running the cross and doing a slip, squat, slip at each end point. That'll get you in the groove. But remember, predictability is your enemy in the ring. Once you hit your stride, change things up. Try a single slip and squat. Imagine your opponent throwing a one-two-three punch combination (a jab, a straight right, and a left hook) and do a slip to the right, a slip to the left, and a squat. If you can think of it, try it. Now is the time to practice your moves—not when you have someone standing in front of you, trying to hit you.

1. Stand in snake position, preferably in front of a full-length mirror.
2. Slip to the right and return to snake position.
3. Squat and return to snake position. Remember to keep your torso vertical—don't bend over—fists up by your chin, and eyes on your imaginary opponent.
4. While still in the squat position, step to the right with your right foot, so your body moves to the other side of the rope. (This is the weave.)
5. Pop, or bob, up into snake position.

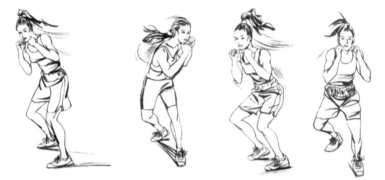

6. Do as many as you can for 3 minutes without losing your form. If you start bending forward or barely squatting, slow down and do it right.

## 1 Minute: Rest

## 15 Minutes: Strength Training

Again, different moves work your muscles in different ways. Variety means that you will burn more calories in a shorter amount of time. Your muscles will be stronger at every angle so you can get off more punches no matter where you or your opponent are standing. Rest for 30 seconds between sets and 1 minute between moves.

## Walking Lunges

*Do 3 sets of 10.*

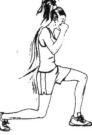

1. Start in the snake position by standing with your feet shoulder-width apart, with your weight centered.
2. Raise both fists to chin level, palms facing inward with your elbows tight to your sides to protect your ribs.
3. Tuck your chin toward your chest and direct your gaze forward at your target, like you're looking through your eyebrows.
4. Keeping your upper body in the snake stance, start at one end of the room and take a long stride forward with the right leg.
5. Bend down so the forward knee is directly over the toes at a 90-degree angle.
6. Raise up and keep repeating while alternating with the other leg until you cross the room.

## Chest Push-ups

*Do 3 sets of 5.*

1. Lie on the floor with your abdomen pressed flat on the floor.
2. Place your hands flat on the floor, beneath your shoulders and shoulder-width apart. Your elbows should be at your sides
3. Push your chest up with your arms, keeping them slightly bent, and hold this position for 10 seconds. Then lower yourself back to the floor.

## Leg Raises

*Do 3 sets of 10.*

1. Lie face up with your back pressed firmly on the floor and your hands behind your head.
2. Raise your legs, with your knees bent slightly, about a foot off the floor and then hold them there.

3. Using just your lower abdominals, tilt your hips and raise your legs higher so that they are not quite at a 90-degree angle. Hold the position for a few seconds, while continuing to breathe.

4. Lower your legs to about a foot off the floor and then hold the position again, before raising them.

## Supermans

*Do 1 set of 3, holding the pose for 10 seconds and resting for 10 seconds in between each rep.*

1. Lie face down on the floor, with your forehead and toes on the floor and your arms extended out in front of your head.

2. Raise your head, chest, arms, and legs off the floor as high as you can without straining yourself—about 3 inches.

3. Hold that position for 3 seconds, then lower your chest, head, arms, legs, and toes to the floor. Repeat.

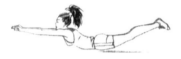

# Parting Shots

Good work—you made it through Week One. You've built a foundation, and you should be feeling tight, your breathing should be a little bit easier, and you may be a little bit sore. You should also be getting used to the way boxing feels—how to hold your hands, how to move your feet, and where to focus your mind. That's good. Now it's time to build on this foundation that you've created. Concentrate on your form and remember everything you've learned as you get ready for your next step—working harder on your strength and stamina, and putting together some punches and more complicated moves. You're strong, you're fit, and you're ready, so let's get going.

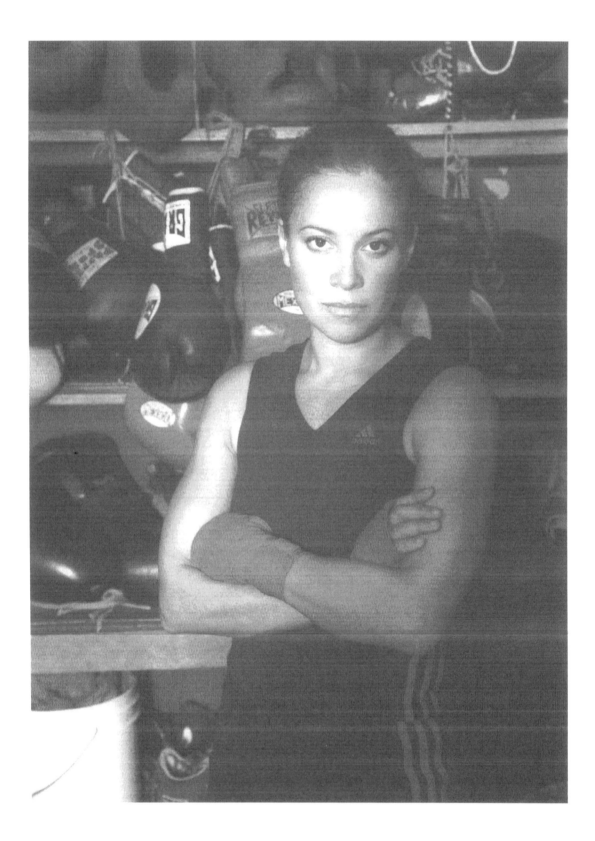

# 7

# Week Two:

## Find Your Style and Strength

Last week was all about setting the groundwork by mastering the footwork. This week, the fun begins. You'll get to start punching!

## Your Fighting Focus: Find Your Style

You've worked on your footwork for a week. Now it is time to add punches to your repertoire and settle into your fighting style. By now, your second week of training, you'll fall into a comfortable style. In the previous chapters, we've been using the terms boxer and fighter interchangeably. But in the sport, there is a difference between the two. A boxer takes advantage of the full range of the ring and uses her footwork to get in close for the attack or out of range to defend herself. She buzzes in and out, like a bee, finding the right place to sting. A fighter uses her body, rather than the ring, as her biggest asset. She stays tight, bobbing and weaving, before stepping into her power punches. She's like a cobra, keeping her body tight, more stationary, and ready to strike.

To avoid the confusion of the terms *boxer* and *fighter,* we'll refer to the two styles as the bee versus the cobra. You've got a 50 percent shot at becoming a bee, and a 50 percent shot at becoming a cobra. Don't worry: This is not a choice you'll have to make. It will come naturally. You don't choose which one you are; your style chooses you.

This week, you'll be mixing last week's footwork—remember the pyramid principle!—with punches, and you'll quickly find what feels natural to you. Last week you did two rounds of jumping rope; this week you'll add another round. The amount of shadowboxing will stay the same to avoid going too hard, too fast. After three rounds-worth of jumping rope, you'll go for a straight three rounds of shadowboxing. Each round of shadowboxing focuses on something different. During the first round, you'll concentrate on moving around the ring and punching, practicing as a boxer. During the second round, you'll shadowbox as a fighter, working on more stationary defenses and close body shots. During the third round, you will focus on the speed of your punches. Don't push them from your shoulder as if your fist is made of lead. Think of your fist as a bullet cutting through the air: Snap each one and draw on the endurance you've built jumping rope to finish strong.

Remember, the point of shadowboxing is to punch and move so many times that your hands know where to go without your head having to think about it. It's more repetition than rocket science. Boxing should become wholly reflexive, as if your body is on autopilot—a fighting machine. That's why we have you practice the same punch over and over and over again, even when you're tired—in fact, especially when you're tired! There will be times when you don't like it, when you feel like you'd rather be in bed. But that isn't going to get you in shape. Push through your fatigue, knowing we're behind you all the way. If you like boxing and you're doing it the right way, you'll enjoy it.

## Your Fitness Focus

This week, you'll make inroads with your endurance, and you'll burn many calories by sandwiching short but intense spurts of cardio between mini-rest periods. The go-and-slow method of training—known as interval training—is *the* quickest way to get fit because it allows you to push your system longer and harder over the course of one workout than you could if you tried to go crazy all at once. It also sends a message to the body that it must prepare itself to handle longer and more intense bouts. The result is that your muscles, including your heart, get stronger, 'your lungs increase their capacity,' and your body actually grows new capillaries, making its delivery of blood and oxygen to your muscles faster and more efficient.

## ★ THE JOY OF ROPE BURN ★

You'll burn far more calories in a shorter period of time by jumping rope than you would by doing practically any other cardio exercise. (Why do you think boxers are so lean?) Check it out: For the next two weeks, you'll jump rope for nine minutes a day to burn between 86 and 116 calories at a pop. Compare that to the number of calories you'd burn doing nine minutes of other types of cardio, using this chart below. All of these calculations are based on a 135-pound woman. If you weigh more, good news—you burn more, too.

| | |
|---|---|
| Jumping Rope | 86–116 calories |
| Yoga | 24 calories |
| Pilates | 29 calories |
| Walking, Moderate Pace | 32 calories |
| Golfing, Carrying Clubs | 43 calories |
| Aerobics | 48 calories |
| Elliptical Trainer | 62 calories |
| Rowing | 67 calories |
| Hiking, Uphill | 72 calories |
| Running, Moderate Pace | 77 calories |
| Biking, Moderate Pace | 77 calories |

# The Workouts: Week Two

## Day One: Work Your Jab
### THE OVERVIEW

Today is going to be a tough day, but it's also going to be the day you fall in love with boxing. You'll jump rope hard for 9 minutes. It's just three minutes more than you're used to, so you can do it if you get your head into it. Visualize the fat melting off your body. Jumping rope, while it's not so glamorous—what in boxing is?—is where you're going to get the biggest body benefits. You'll burn off fat and uncover muscle tone you never knew you had. And where you don't have muscle tone, you'll build it through your daily strength training. You'll also start punching for the first time today. You'll start by just jabbing and moving. Then, you'll add defensive maneuvers alongside your jabs, and finally you'll work up to throwing a few combinations in rapid succession. You are going to feel amazing after today's workout. Tired, but amazing.

## What You're Going to Do Today:
### WEEK TWO, DAY ONE

| 9 Minutes: | Jump Rope |
|---|---|
| | 3 Minutes @ Level 3–4 |
| | 1 Minute @ Level 5–6 |
| | 1 Minute @ Level 7–8 |
| | 1 Minute @ Level 5–6 |
| | 3 Minutes @ Level 3–4 |
| 1 Minute: | Rest |

| | |
|---|---|
| 3 Minutes: | Shadowboxing |
| | *Step + Jab + Move Sideways* |
| | *Double Jab + Circle* |
| | *Jab to the Body + Jab to the Chin + Move* |
| 1 Minute: | Rest |
| 3 Minutes: | Shadowboxing |
| | *Duck + Jab* |
| | *Jab + Slip Right + Slip Left* |
| | *1 + 2 + Duck* |
| 1 Minute: | Rest |
| 3 Minutes: | Shadowboxing |
| | *1 + 2 + 3* |
| | *1 + 2 + 1 + 2* |
| | *Jab to the Body + 1 + 2 + 3* |
| 1 Minute: | Rest |
| 15 Minutes: | Strength Training |
| | *Jump Squats: 3 sets of 10* |
| | *Alligator Push-ups: 3 sets of 8* |
| | *Side Scissors: 3 sets of 12* |
| | *Crunches: 3 sets of 12* |

# The Details

## 9 Minutes: Jump Rope

Warm-up for 3 minutes at a steady level 3–4 pace. Ramp up your intensity, pushing yourself to a level 5–6 for 1 minute. Now dial it up once more, to a level 7–8, and hold it for 1 minute. Catch your breath again for a minute at level 5–6. Cool down for 3 minutes at a level 3–4. Remember, now that you've gotten a hang of jumping rope, feel free to do whatever it takes to keep your mind focused. If you want to run in place over the rope, go ahead. Like heel skipping? Do it. Want to get fancy and add a few crossovers into your regimen, say every time you change your speed, that's totally up to you. Feel free to vary your jump-roping style as often as you like today and throughout the rest of the workout.

## 1 Minute: Rest

Congratulate yourself for going the longest you've ever gone on the rope, and then start thinking why you're working so hard for yourself. Do you want to change your body? You are. Do you want to learn to fight? You are. Do you want to have more energy? You do already.

## 3 Minutes: Shadowboxing

This round will be your first chance to get a feel for the different fighting styles. Remember there are two. The bee buzzes in and out, finding the right place to sting. She moves around the ring to throw off her opponent. The cobra keeps her body tight, more stationary, and ready to strike. In this round, try your hand as a bee by taking advantage of all the space around you. Make that your goal today and focus on snapping your punches and landing them exactly where you want them to go. When you jab, you should be aiming for that sweet spot between your opponent's chin and chest. (That way, if she ducks too slowly, you'll still hit her nose.) Below are the moves to practice during round one. You can do them in any order and for any length of time. Just be sure to do each one often enough so that you feel equally comfortable with all three moves by the end of the round.

## Make the Most of Your Combinations

This week you're doing combinations of punches for the first time. It's important to do them correctly; otherwise, you'll get hit. Here are a few things you *must* remember anytime you string more than one punch together.

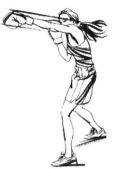

1. In most cases, start with a jab as your first punch. In a real fight, the most successful combinations begin with a jab. Although you can mix it up, in general, this punch will set you up for the next one without leaving you too open to a counterpunch.

2. Always return to the snake position between punches. You never want both of your fists away from your face at one time.

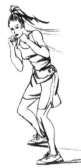

3. Use speed, not power. If you try and put too much power behind one punch, you may throw yourself off balance, leaving yourself open and unable to throw the next one. So be quick and on target rather than extra strong.

4. Know your next move. Don't spend time thinking *What's my next punch?*

5. Keep your weight centered on both feet, and stay on the balls of your feet.

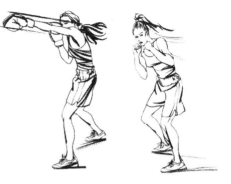

◆ **Step + Jab + Move Sideways:** Start in snake position, and immediately after stepping forward with your left foot, snap—don't push—your jab. Then move from side to side.

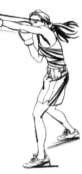

◆ **Double Jab + Circle:** Throw your first jab, return to the snake position, and throw your second jab right away. Do it as fast as you can without sacrificing your form. You don't want to give your opponent time to think or respond. As soon as you make (imaginary) impact on the second jab, bring your fist back and start circling your opponent. Reverse directions quickly and frequently, and double jab again.

◆ **Jab to the Body + Jab to the Chin + Move:** Start by squatting, keeping your back straight. Deliver a jab to the body, then pop back into the snake position. With the same hand, jab your opponent's chin. Before she can muster a response, move to the side. This is the perfect move for when your opponent's stomach is open, or you've just ducked her hook. Be an efficient player: You're already at eye-level to her navel, so you may as well hit her on the way back up.

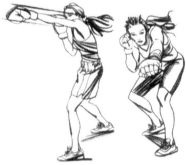

## 1 Minute: Rest

## 3 Minutes: Shadowboxing

Try this round as a cobra, rather than a bee, by trying moves you'd use if you stuck close to your opponent. You'll also bring your straight right out for the first time today, and it is going to feel so satisfying. Here are your 3 moves for round two. Mix them up and, we can't say it enough, remember the pyramid principle! Just because you're taking this round as a cobra doesn't mean you should be flat on your feet. Along with the punches from today's first round of shadowboxing, stay on your toes by adding some of last week's footwork like bobbing, weaving, and circling.

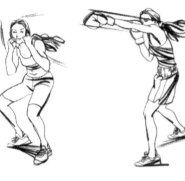

◆ **Duck + Jab:** When you duck a punch, you want to respond immediately with a counter; the faster you can do it, the more effective it'll be because you'll be more likely to catch your opponent either out of position or off balance. Duck quickly, keeping your back straight, and as soon as you return to snake position, throw a jab to her chin. By the way, this move is a great butt, thigh, and shoulder toner.

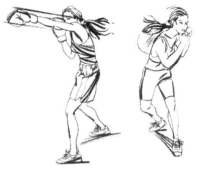

- **Jab + Slip Right + Slip Left:** Since the jab is the most frequently thrown punch in boxing, it's important to be able to both throw it and slip it in one fluid movement. Starting in snake position, throw a jab with your left hand. Return to snake position and then turn first to the right, then to the left. Always keep your eyes on your opponent and your fists up to protect your chin.

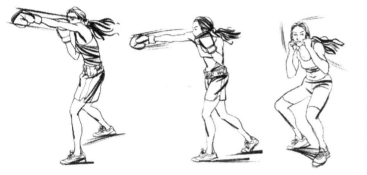

- **1 + 2 + Duck:** A 1-2 punch is shorthand for a jab followed immediately by a straight right. After you throw the sequence, duck down to avoid an imaginary hook. Remember, keep your eyes on your opponent at all times. When you're low, that means you're looking up at her through your eyebrows.

## 1 Minute: Rest

## 3 Minutes: Shadowboxing

You've worked on your form during the past two rounds today. Now, it's time to work on your speed. Not only will this drill help you have fast hands, but it'll also build your stamina and endurance. At the end of every round, you need to be able to find and summon that last drop of energy hidden deep inside you. This is what you will practice in this round.

You're going to work on stringing 3 punches together and throwing your first 4-punch combinations. During the first 50 seconds of each minute of this round, practice moving and punching. During the last 10 seconds of each minute of this round, practice throwing a flurry of punches—anything you've learned to this point—in rapid succession. You can do this. You know the punches and footwork well enough to pull this off. It's about having faith in yourself and your training. Just don't stop. Don't pause to think. Don't hesitate.

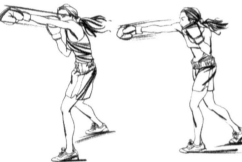

◆ **1 + 2 + 1 + 2:** You've already practiced the 1-2 punch, which is the jab followed by the straight right. Now practice throwing 2-1-2 back to back for your first 4-punch combination.

◆ **1 + 2 + 3:** If you spot an opening, this is one of the royal sequences you'll want to throw. It's a match ender: the jab, followed by the straight right, and then a quick left hook to the chin. During your left hook, remember to pivot your front foot to get the power behind your punch. It comes from your hips. After you complete the sequence, try moving side to side, or circling, or ducking. You always want your next few moves lined up before you finish what you're doing, so you can lead the fight.

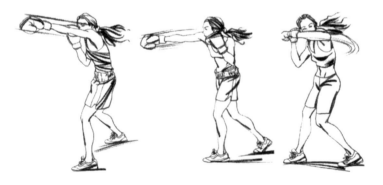

◆ **Jab to the Body + 1 + 2 + 3:** Drop down into a squat to deliver a left jab to the body, and then spring up and punish your opponent with a jab, straight right, and left hook combination.

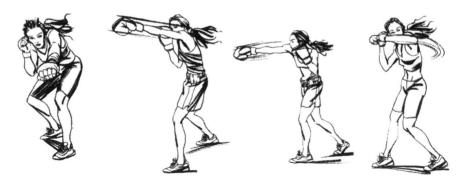

## 1 Minute: Rest

## 15 Minutes: Strength Training

This week, you'll increase your reps of each exercise. And as you did last week, rest 30 seconds between each set and 1 minute between each move.

*Jump Squats*

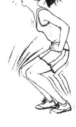

*Do 3 sets of 10.*

*Alligator Push-Ups*

*Do 3 sets of 8. Use your knees, if you need to.*
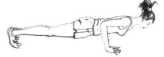

*Side Scissors*

Do 3 sets of 12.

*Crunches*

*Do 3 sets of 12.*

# Day Two: Master Placement
## THE OVERVIEW

Try to workout in front of a mirror today, and use your reflection, not for observing your own form, but for target practice. Obviously, stay out of reach, but when punching, aim for your own, say, chin or ribs. Accuracy, not power, will always win out in the ring. Use the same set of rounds for the shadowboxing drills this week: Approach round one as a boxer, round two as a fighter, and round three as a speed demon. Every day we're going to expect more from you, but every day, you're also going to get fitter, which means you'll be able to do more, too.

# What You're Going to Do Today:
## WEEK TWO, DAY TWO

| | |
|---|---|
| 9 Minutes: | Jump Rope |
| | 3 Minutes @ Level 3–4 |
| | 1 Minute @ Level 5–6 |
| | 1 Minute @ Level 7–8 |
| | 1 Minute @ Level 5–6 |
| | 1 Minute @ Level 7–8 |
| | 2 Minutes @ Level 3–4 |
| 1 Minute: | Rest |
| 3 Minutes: | Shadowboxing |
| | Jab + Step + Hook |
| | Jab to the Body + Jab + Jab to the Body |
| | 1 + 2 + Left Hook to the Body |
| 1 Minute: | Rest |

| 3 Minutes: | Shadowboxing |
| --- | --- |
| | *Left Hook to the Body + Left Hook to the Body* |
| | *Right Uppercut + Left Uppercut* |
| | *Straight Right to the Body + Left Hook* |

| 1 Minute: | Rest |
| --- | --- |

| 3 Minutes: | Shadowboxing |
| --- | --- |
| | *Left Hook + Right Uppercut + Left Hook* |
| | *1 + 2 + Left Hook to the Body +* |
| | *Right Hook to the Body* |
| | *Jab + Right Uppercut + Left Hook + Left Hook* |

| 1 Minute: | Rest |
| --- | --- |

| 15 Minutes: | Strength Training |
| --- | --- |
| | *Bicycle: 3 sets of 50* |
| | *Bow: 1 set of 3, 15-second holds* |
| | *Triangle Push-ups: 3 sets of 5* |
| | *Flutter Kicks: 3 sets of 15* |

# The Details

### 9 Minutes: Jump Rope

Today, you're going to squeeze in one more minute of intense rope jumping work, but it won't feel so hard because we're building in mini-rest periods between each vigorous bout. So here's the deal: Warm up, as usual, for 3 minutes at a level 3–4. Then, for the next 4 minutes, alternate 1 minute of moderate intensity rope jumping (level 5–6) with 1 minute of high intensity rope jumping (level 7–8). Recover with 2 minutes at level 3–4.

### 1 Minute: Rest

Good job on the jump rope. Now, decide what you're fighting for today. Flat abs? More confidence? It's up to you.

### 3 Minutes: Shadowboxing

Don't worry too much about the speed of your punches during this round. Instead, focus on flowing smoothly from one punch to the next and landing each one exactly where you intend to. Use your reflection to check your placement.

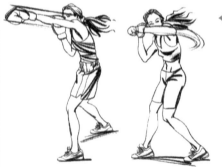

◆ **Jab + Step + Hook:** It's exactly as it sounds. Distract your opponent with a jab to the chin, then take a quick step forward toward your opponent. By the time she recovers her vision, you'll have already moved in close for a left hook.

◆ **Jab to the Body + Jab + Jab to the Body:** Don't get lazy, or you'll start throwing the punch before your body moves into proper position. You may as well be throwing wet noodles at your opponent.

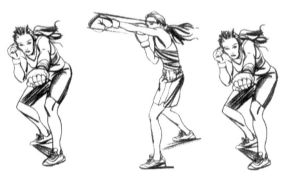

You're not going to have any power behind you. Do it right or put the book down, walk away, and come back when you're ready to do it right. Squat first, *then* jab to the body; return to snake position, then jab to the chin; squat, then jab to the body again.

- ◆ **1 + 2 + Left Hook to the Body:** Keep your weight evenly balanced during your jab and straight right so you can stay centered as you squat down to throw the left hook into the body. Remember, on the left hook to the body, move your fist in *and* upward.

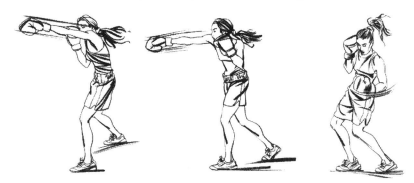

## 1 Minute: Rest

## 3 Minutes: Shadowboxing

When your opponent pushes or leans close to you (or hopefully staggers close to you), you want to be prepared to respond with a rapid succession of body shots. Here are three good two-punch series on which you can always rely.

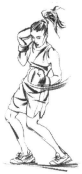

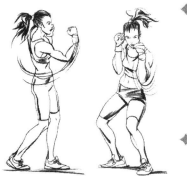

- ◆ **Left Hook to the Body + Left Hook to the Body:** Don't forget to keep your right fist up to protect your chin from a sneaky left hook. Remember your angle on the left hook to the body: in and up.

- ◆ **Right Uppercut + Left Uppercut:** If your opponent ever tilts forward—maybe she's getting lazy in her body setup—

her chin is just hanging out in the open waiting to receive your uppercuts. Go for it. Uppercut punches are especially good for strengthening your abs.

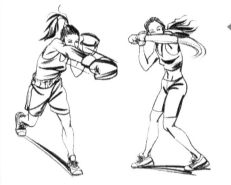

◆ **Straight Right to the Body + Left Hook:** This will push your opponent away. Squat for your straight right to the body, and then spring back up for a quick left hook to the chin. Keep your eyes on your opponent at all times. If she falls back after your first punch, you may need to take a step forward so you can land your hook. Practice that variation, too.

1 Minute: Rest

## 3 Minutes: Shadowboxing

These combinations can be tricky, which is why you need to do them over and over again until your muscles automatically memorize the movements. During this round, work on your speed of delivery again. Work at 50 to 60 percent of your full capacity the first 50 seconds of each minute, and then finish off with a 10-second flurry of combinations. In other words, you should be breathing hard, but still able to have a conversation without gasping for air.

◆ **Left Hook + Right Uppercut + Left Hook:** Your feet are going to pivot 3 times during this sequence: First, your front foot will turn in for the hook, then your back will turn in for the uppercut, and then your front foot will turn in again for the left hook.

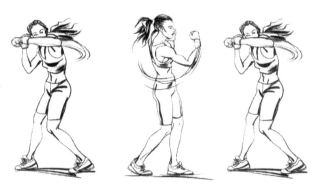

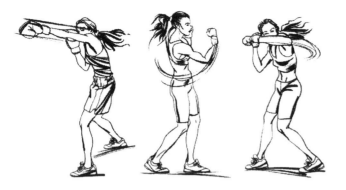

- **Jab + Right Uppercut + Left Hook + Left Hook:** This sequence is particularly effective when your opponent gets too cozy.

- **1 + 2 + Left Hook to the Body + Right Hook to the Body:** Squat down, don't lean, for the body shots, and don't forget that the form for the left and right hooks are different. Throw a left hook with your palm facing down and your thumb facing toward you. But when you throw a right hook, pretend like you're throwing a beer mug: Your palm should be facing you and your thumb facing upward. Again, don't forget to pivot both feet. You'll protect your knees and find more power.

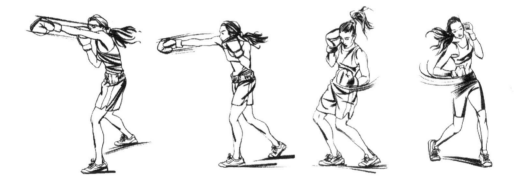

## 1 Minute: Rest

## 15 Minutes: Strength Training

Do a few more reps today. Rest for 30 seconds between sets and 1 minute between moves.

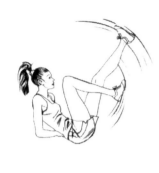

## Bicycle

*Do 3 sets of 50.*

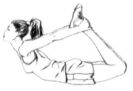

## Bow

*Do 1 set of 3, holding the pose for 15 seconds and resting for 10 seconds between each rep.*

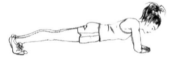

## Triangle Push-ups

*Do 3 sets of 5. Use your knees if need be.*

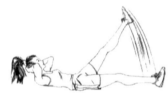

## Flutter Kicks

*Do 3 sets of 15.*

# Day Three: Learn Some Surprises

Head into the weekend knowing that you're going to feel excellent after today's workout, which includes your most challenging cardio rope-work yet. (Don't worry; you don't have to jump rope for a longer time, just a little bit harder.) This is the same format for your shadowboxing as the rest of week: Round one includes a few top combinations for boxers who make use of their space; round two includes some body shots, perfect for infighting; and round three is your chance to work at some more surprising combinations at serious speeds. That's where your newfound endurance will start helping you out. Remember to add any of the other moves you've practiced so far into any of these rounds whenever you feel so inspired. At this point, you should be perfecting your punches and your moves. Pay close attention to your form.

After today, take a few days off and feel proud of yourself for working so hard. You're halfway to being ring-ready, or depending on how you look at it, twice as ready to spar as you were two weeks ago. You're putting everything together and keeping your head in it. You're looking like a fighter.

## What You're Going to Do Today:
WEEK TWO, DAY THREE

| 9 Minutes: | Jump Rope | |
|---|---|---|
| | 3 Minutes | @ Level 3–4 |
| | 30 Seconds | @ Level 5–6 |
| | 1 Minute | @ Level 7–8 |
| | 30 Seconds | @ Level 5–6 |
| | 1 Minute | @ Level 7–8 |
| | 30 Seconds | @ Level 5–6 |
| | 1 Minute | @ Level 7–8 |
| | 1.5 Minutes | @ Level 3–4 |

| | |
|---|---|
| 1 Minute: | Rest |
| 3 Minutes: | Shadowboxing<br>*Jab + Jab + Left Hook*<br>*Jab + Right Hook + Left Hook*<br>*Jab + Step + Left Hook + Right Cross* |
| 1 Minute: | Rest |
| 3 Minutes: | Shadowboxing<br>*Right Uppercut + Right Cross + Left Hook*<br>*Right Uppercut + Left Hook to the Body + Straight Right*<br>*Left Uppercut + Right Uppercut + Left Hook + Straight Right* |
| 1 Minute: | Rest |
| 3 Minutes: | Shadowboxing<br>*Jab + Jab + Left Uppercut + Right Cross*<br>*1 + 2 + Left Hook to the Body + Right Cross*<br>*Jab + Right Cross + Jab + Left Hook* |
| 1 Minute: | Rest |
| 15 Minutes: | Strength Training<br>*Walking Lunges: 3 sets of 12*<br>*Chest Push-Ups: 3 sets of 8*<br>*Leg Raises: 3 sets of 12*<br>*Supermans: 1 set of 3, holding for 15 seconds* |

# The Details

## 9 Minutes: Jump Rope

Limit your intense spurts to a minute, like you've been doing already, but this time, reduce the rest periods between them. So, warm up for 3 minutes at level 3–4. For the next 30 seconds, increase your intensity to a level 5–6. Then, for the next minute, go hard at a level 7–8. Repeat that sequence 2 more times (for a total of 3 more minutes), before cooling down for a minute and a half at level 3–4.

## 1 Minute: Rest

Have you noticed that you're doing things you never dreamed of only two weeks ago! Revel in that for a moment and think about what you're going to be able to do (and how you're going to look) in another two weeks.

## 3 Minutes: Shadowboxing

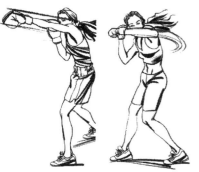

Don't forget to make full use of your space. Make your opponent go exactly where you want her to go. In fact, start this round with some movement: circle a bit, advance, and retreat. Once you feel loose, start throwing the following punches:

◆ **Jab + Jab + Left Hook:** A double jab is often a setup for a straight right. Throw your opponent off by skipping over it and moving directly to a left hook.

◆ **Jab + Right Hook + Left Hook:** Try this combination slowly at first, making sure your right palm is facing you during your right hook and your left palm is facing down during your left hook.

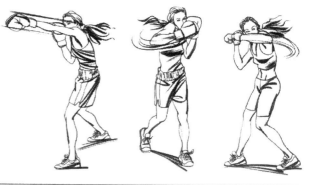

◆ **Jab + Step + Left Hook + Right Cross:** You've already practiced this combination once before, but this time, you're adding a power punch—the right cross—as a finale. Don't get caught flat-footed when you're through. Keep moving: Advance, retreat, circle, bob and weave, and/or move from side to side.

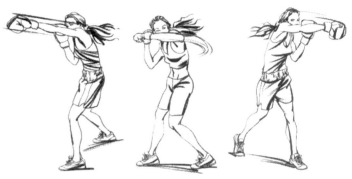

### 1 Minute: Rest

### 3 Minutes: Shadowboxing

It practically takes longer to call these sequences than it does to actually deliver them. As you throw the body shots, think about how you'd defend yourself against them. Defend your body with an elbow block or by moving out of the way, and defend your face with a duck or slip.

◆ **Right Uppercut + Right Cross + Left Hook:** This sequence will only work when you really nail the right uppercut; otherwise, it'll take too long to set-up for your right cross. During your uppercut, strike upward, as if you're going to punch through the ceiling. Ideally, you'll punch your opponent right under her chin, causing her head to fall back and her face to open up for a pain-inducing right cross.

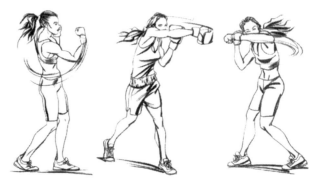

- **Right Uppercut + Left Hook to the Body + Straight Right:** Get your angles right on these punches to make them most effective. Move your fist directly upward on the uppercut, at a 45-degree angle in *and* up on the left hook to the body, and parallel to the floor on the straight right.

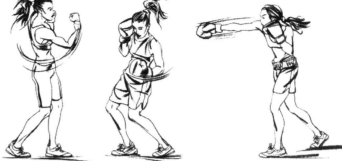

- **Left Uppercut + Right Uppercut + Left Hook + Straight Right:** Do them enough, and the 2 uppercuts will work wonders for your abs, especially on those hard-to-tone obliques. All of the above punches come in combinations where the jab is thrown first.

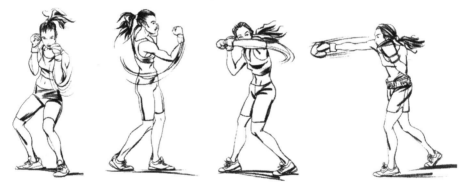

## 1 Minute: Rest

## 3 Minutes: Shadowboxing

This is your speed round. Finish each minute by going hard for 10 seconds. Today, try ducking between each combination and see how many you can get through before time is up.

◆ **Jab + Jab + Left Up-percut + Right Cross:** Tease with your left; finish with your right.

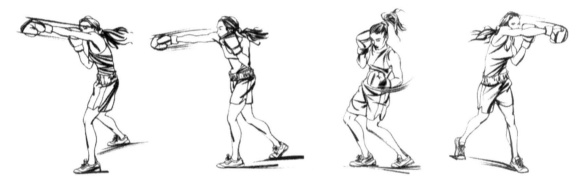

◆ **1 + 2 + Left Hook to the Body + Right Cross:** If you nail this sequence, you will be wearing a grin all weekend. It is so satisfying to deliver.

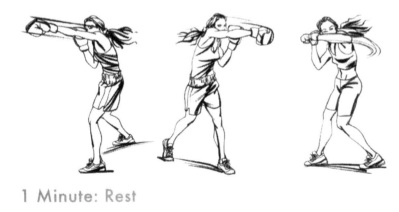

◆ **Jab + Right Cross + Jab + Left Hook:** Use your jabs to distract and/or blind your opponent, so you can sneak in 2 power punches—the right cross and the left hook.

1 Minute: Rest

## 15 Minutes: Strength Training

This is the same deal as the previous days: Rest for 30 seconds between sets and 1 minute between moves. For an added challenge, hold light weights in each hand during the walking lunges.

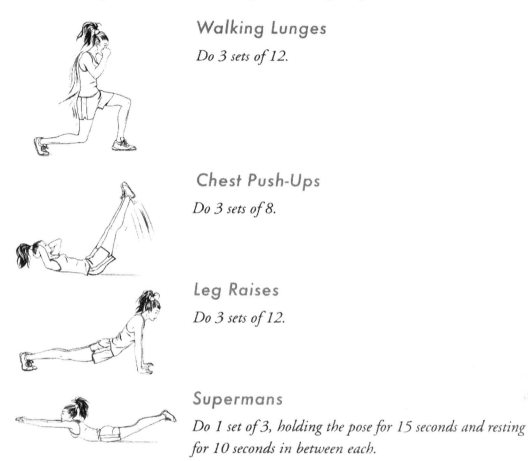

### Walking Lunges

*Do 3 sets of 12.*

### Chest Push-Ups

*Do 3 sets of 8.*

### Leg Raises

*Do 3 sets of 12.*

### Supermans

*Do 1 set of 3, holding the pose for 15 seconds and resting for 10 seconds in between each.*

# Parting Shots

Great work. You've mastered some complicated combinations, improved your footwork, and been versatile enough to go back and forth between different styles. Best of all, you've got half of this workout behind you. But you've got the other half ahead, so keep going. Now's not the time to start slacking off. Stay strong and focused on your form. Prove to yourself that you've got what it takes to be a real champion.

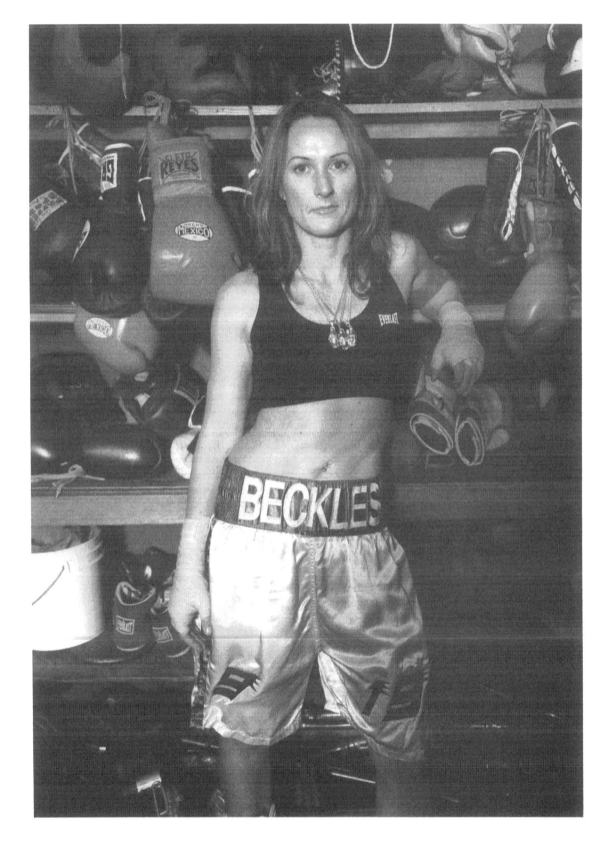

# 8

# Week Three:

## Counterpunch

Congratulations! You hit the halfway point, and you should be feeling better than ever. This week's workout is both physically and mentally more challenging than last week's, but it's exactly what you've been working toward. You are well-prepared to begin counterpunching, which takes quickness, concentration, and stamina. The workout so far has sharpened both your mental and physical reflexes, so we know you're ready.

### Your Fighting Focus:

You already know how to move and how to put basic punches together. Now, it's time to add strategy to the mix. It's as important to know *when* to throw certain combinations as it is to know how to throw them. You always want to be leading the fight. You want to know what punches you plan to throw three, four, or five moves before you actually throw them. That is every boxer's ideal situation. But things in the ring don't always work out as planned, so it's crucial to learn how to wrest control of the match back when you're getting pummeled. You've got to study your opponent's patterns, even as they're landing on your jaw. Learn which combinations she falls back on time after time—every boxer has a few favorites—and then deliver the appropriate response. Reading her punches and answering them with a specifically chosen retort is called counterpunching. It's the art of turning your defense into offense.

## Your Fitness Focus:

Last week, you used intervals to build your endurance. This week, you'll still train with intervals, but your goal now is to stretch each intense bout a bit longer. Not only will you burn more calories, but also your body will adjust to the harder, longer workload, making your heart, your lungs, and your muscles (especially your thighs, calves, and buttocks) stronger and fitter. In fighting terms, last week, you were conditioned enough to eke out a final flurry of punches at the end of each the round. By the end of this week, you'll be able to wage several sustained attacks on your opponent throughout the round without feeling like each is a last-gasp effort. By the end of this week, you'll also notice that your clothes will start to fit a little looser, and you'll begin to see some real definition in your upper arms.

## ★ REMINDER: THE PYRAMID PRINCIPLE ★

This week, you'll be working on counterpunching and combinations with more punches. So the pyramid principle is key, especially if you find that you're pausing too much because you don't know what to do. You shouldn't have "dead air time." New skills should not replace the old ones; they should build on them so that you have a full inventory of moves and punches to practice. In other words, just because you're working on five-punch combinations, it doesn't mean you should forget the basics like bobbing and weaving or one-two. The basics are just as important to your skill set as the more complicated combinations, so don't leave them behind. No matter what you're working on, advance, retreat, and circle between sequences.

# The Workouts: Week Three

## Day One: How to Counter the One-Two

### THE OVERVIEW

You're going to burn more calories today than you ever have before. Your jumping rope will last three minutes longer, and you'll push each high-intensity interval for 30 seconds longer. The higher you jump, the harder the workout becomes for all of your muscles, especially your legs and heart. So, if you get tired, either reduce your rope speed or your vertical jump. Remember to switch things up to keep it interesting, too. Put on some music. Try skipping backward. Incorporate crossovers each time you switch speed.

Today's shadowboxing workout requires a bit more imagination than you're used to in the past. Since you're not actually sparring or working with a trainer in person, you've got to visualize your opponent throwing punches, which you're going to counter. You'll go for three rounds again—the same as last week. During the first round, you'll work on counters to your opponent's jab to your chin and body. During the second round, you'll learn counters to her straight rights to your chin and your body. Picture her fists coming toward you, and respond with rapid sharpness. You'll be tired after twelve minutes of jumping rope, but if you shadowbox sluggishly, it's not worth it. You're just going to make yourself look bad, and you're not going to develop the reflexes you'll eventually need in the ring. Round three is a speed drill again. You'll launch a longer, more sustained attack, aimed at building your endurance. When you're through, bang out some more strength-training moves—a few more reps of each than last week—to build some definition. You'll have burned off lots of fat by now. The strength exercises will give you some contour, so you won't look like a worm.

# What You're Going to Do Today:

| | |
|---|---|
| 12 Minutes: | Jump Rope |
| | *3 Minutes @ Level 3–4* |
| | *30 Seconds @ Level 5–6* |
| | *1.5 Minutes @ Level 7–8* |
| | *30 Seconds @ Level 5–6* |
| | *1.5 Minutes @ Level 7–8* |
| | *30 Seconds @ Level 5–6* |
| | *1.5 Minutes @ Level 7–8* |
| | *3 Minutes @ Level 3–4* |
| 1 Minute: | Rest |
| 3 Minutes: | Shadowboxing: Counter Straight Left |
| | *Duck + Step + Straight Right to the Body + Left Hook* |
| | *Slip Right + Right Hook + Duck + Left Uppercut* |
| | *Elbow Block + Left Upper cut + Right Overhand* |
| 1 Minute: | Rest |
| 3 Minutes: | Shadowboxing: Counter ingStraight Rights |
| | *Duck + Left Hook + Right Cross* |
| | *Step Right + Double Jab* |
| | *Elbow Block + Right Uppercut + Left Hook to the Body + Left Hook* |
| 1 Minute: | Rest |

| | |
|---|---|
| 3 Minutes: | Shadowboxing 15 seconds/60 seconds |
| | *Triple Jab + Straight Right* |
| | *1 + 2 + 3 + 4* |
| | *Jab + Straight Right + Left Hook + Straight Right* |
| 1 Minute: | Rest |
| 15 Minutes: | Strength Training |
| | *Jump Squats:* 3 sets of 12 |
| | *Alligator Push-Ups:* 3 sets of 10 |
| | *Side Scissors:* 3 sets of 15 |
| | *Twist Crunches:* 3 sets of 15 |

# The Details

## 12 Minutes: Jump Rope

Warm up for 3 minutes at a steady level 3–4 pace. Then, raise it up for 30 seconds to a level 5–6, and then let loose at a level 7–8 for a minute and a half. Repeat the sequence 2 more times, before cooling down for 2 minutes at a level 3–4. Remember, you can jump rope any way you please, so long as you're working your heart and feet.

## 1 Minute: Rest

Take a moment to think about how far you've come since day one and how the way you look and feel has changed. Picture yourself in the ring, sparring against an opponent, and imagine how you're going to defend yourself against her.

## 3 Minutes: Shadowboxing: Countering Lefts

This round is all about countering the jab and jab to the body. As you know, the point of your opponent's jab is to throw you off balance, divert your attention from the next punch coming, or draw your hands away from your face. So, to defend yourself, you want to move first, to clear your line of vision, maintain your balance, and maybe throw her balance off. Then, you want to counter right away, before she draws her hand back in a protective position.

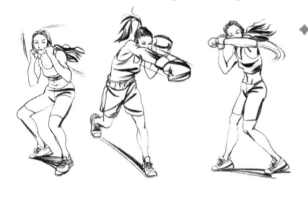

◆ **Duck + Step + Straight Right to the Body + Left Hook:** If you duck a jab and counter quick enough, your opponent's entire abdomen should be wide open because her left arm is extended and her right hand is next to her chin. Take advantage of this opening by taking a step toward her and delivering a powerful right. Spring back up to snake position and finish it off with a left hook.

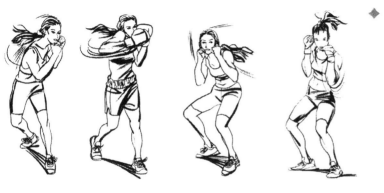

♦ **Slip Right + Right Hook + Duck + Left Uppercut:** After you slip a jab to the right, causing your opponent's fist to pass behind your head, your hips will be in perfect cocked position to pivot sharply and power a right hook. Often, your opponent will follow a missed jab with another jab. You can duck this one and counter from the other side with a left uppercut. She won't know what hit her.

♦ **Elbow Block (right) + Left Uppercut + Right Overhand:** The jab to 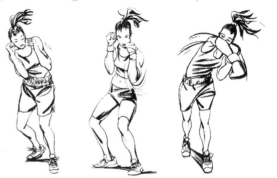 the body is a teasing punch. Its purpose is to nag your hands down to open up your face for a punch. Since there's very little power behind the jab to the body, you can easily block it with your right elbow, which will leave your face well-protected. Counter with a surprise under-over sequence: a left uppercut and a right overhand.

## 1 Minute: Rest

## 3 Minutes: Shadowboxing: Countering Straight Rights

You can only take so many rights to the chin or body, which is why it's important to be quick on the defense and respond aggressively. The fighter who relies too heavily on her right is more likely to be strong than well-conditioned. She counts on her power, not her stamina or speed, to bring down her opponent. The key to winning matches against this type of fighter is to make her move and wear her down, and if that doesn't work, keep hitting her in the arms, until she's too tired to raise them.

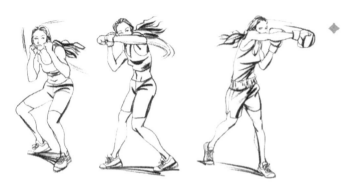

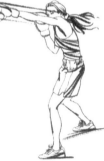

**Duck + Left Hook + Right Cross:** Once you duck the right, the left hook makes for a natural counter, especially if she untucks her chin from her chest. Finish with a right cross.

◆ **Step Right + Double Jab:** A quick step to the right will put your left lead right between her hands. Counter with your quickest, sharpest double jab, while keeping your right hand on guard against a left hook.

◆ **Elbow Block (left) + Right Uppercut + Left Hook to the Body + Left Hook:** It only takes one good straight right to the body to knock you off your top game. This punch steals your wind, which is why you need a defense at the ready. If you can, move out of the way, block the straight right with your left elbow, and catch her chin with a right uppercut. Then, tire out her right side with a left hook to the body (or arm) and a left hook to the chin.

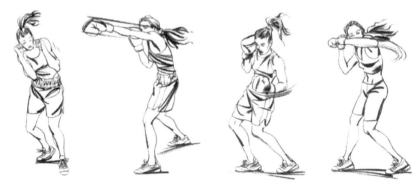

1 Minute: Rest

## 3 Minutes: Shadowboxing

Here's more speed-work for today to help you build fast hands and more endurance. During this round, you'll learn a few new combinations. Find your rhythm for the first 45 seconds of each minute, and then bang the combinations out in rapid succession (without sacrificing your form or targeting) for the last 15 seconds of every minute. This isn't easy: You're going to have to call on your reserves of endurance and concentration. But we wouldn't ask you to do anything you're not ready for. You've trained hard to this point, and you can do this. Show off a little bit; make this fun.

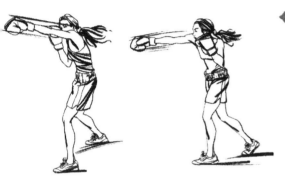

♦ **Triple Jab + Straight Right:** If your opponent is trying to close in on you, the triple jab will give you some space and put your opponent on her back foot, especially if you've got a longer reach. (Depending on your proximity, you may have to step in before each punch.) Then knock her down with a straight right.

♦ **1-2-3-4:** This is *the* classic combination: A jab, followed by a straight right, a left hook, and a right uppercut. Keep it in your back pocket, ready to pull out at any time.

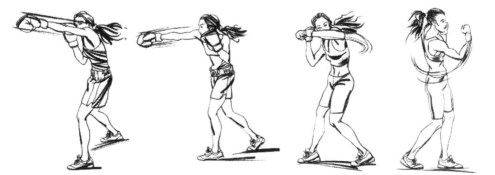

◆ **Jab + Straight Right + Left Hook + Straight Right:** This is a variation on the last sequence, only you'll surprise your opponent with a straight right, rather than a right uppercut. You'll learn something key here: Lots of fighters get into predictable patterns. If you find yourself resorting to the same combinations, it's nice to at least have some unexpected finishes on expected beginnings.

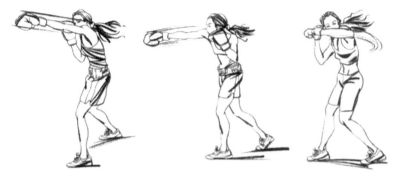

## 1 Minute: Rest

## 15 Minutes: Strength Training

This week, you'll increase your reps of each exercise once again, and you'll also decrease the amount of rest time between each move. It'll keep your heart rate elevated, and you'll burn more calories. Rest 30 seconds both between each set and between each move.

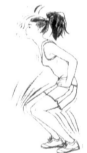

### Jump Squats

*Do 3 sets of 12.*

### Alligator Push-ups

*Do 3 sets of 10. Use your knees if you need to.*

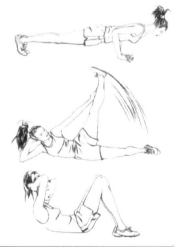

### Side Scissors

*Do 3 sets of 15.*

### Crunches

*Do 3 sets of 15.*

# Day Two: Countering Hooks
## THE OVERVIEW

The key to defending yourself against and countering hooks is speed. You've got to read the punch early by keeping the corner of your eye on your opponent's elbows. As soon as you spot her elbow moving up and away from her ribs—even if her fists haven't yet moved away from her face—you know she's going to throw a hook. It's the only punch that requires your forearm to turn parallel to the ground. When you see her elbow flying, make a decision: Either step in and counterpunch before she has a chance to pull off her hook or duck, and force her to miss and lose her balance.

# What You're Going to Do Today:
## WEEK THREE, DAY TWO

| | |
|---|---|
| 12 Minutes: | Jump Rope |
| | *2 Minutes   @ Level 3–4* |
| | *30 Seconds @ Level 5–6* |
| | *2 Minutes   @ Level 7–8* |
| | *30 Seconds @ Level 5–6* |
| | *2 Minutes   @ Level 7–8* |
| | *30 Seconds @ Level 5–6* |
| | *2 Minutes   @ Level 7–8* |
| | *2.5 Minutes @ Level 3–4* |
| 1 Minute: | Rest |
| 3 Minutes: | Shadowboxing: Countering Left Hooks |
| | *Step + Jab + Right Hook to the Body* |
| | *Step + Straight Right + Left Hook + Right* |
| | *Uppercut + Left Hook* |
| | *Elbow Block (Right) + 1 + 2* |

| 1 Minute: | Rest |
|---|---|
| 3 Minutes: | Shadowboxing: Counter Right Hooks |
| | *Duck + 1 + 2 to the Body* |
| | *Step + Jab + Straight Right to the Body + Left Hook* |
| | *Elbow Block (Left) + Right Overhand + Left Hook* |
| 1 Minute: | Rest |
| 3 Minutes: | Shadowboxing |
| | *Jab + Right Cross + Jab* |
| | *Straight Right to the Body + Left Hook to the Body + Right Hook + Left Hook* |
| | *Jab + Right Uppercut + Straight Right* |
| 1 Minute: | Rest |
| 15 Minutes: | Strength Training |
| | *Bicycle: 3 sets of 75* |
| | *Bow: 1 set of 3, 20 second holds* |
| | *Triangle Push-ups: 3 sets of 8* |
| | *Flutter Kicks: 3 sets of 20* |

# The Details

## 12 Minutes: Jump Rope

After a 2-minute warm-up (level 3–4), crank it up a notch to a level 5–6 for 30 seconds. Then, open it up to a level 7–8 for a full 2 minutes by varying either your speed or vertical jump. Repeat 2 more times. Cool down at a level 3–4 for the remaining 2.5 minutes.

## 1 Minute: Rest

Walk around slowly. Relax, take deep breaths, and get loose. Revel in your progress. Then get your head set for a fierce round of shadowboxing. Keep the pyramid principle in mind. During the next few rounds, you always want to be moving around and incorporating any punches you can think of between the new combinations that you're learning.

## 3 Minutes: Shadowboxing: Countering Left Hooks

Today you're going to practice counterpunching against a left hook. Good timing, depth perception, and practice are critical.

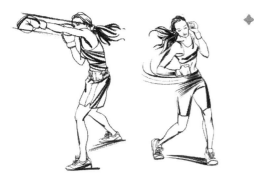

◆ **Step + Jab + Right Hook to the Body:** The jab is always quicker to get off than a hook, so if you read the hook early enough, you can step in and to the left and snap your jab, keeping your right hand up on the defensive. That'll throw your opponent off balance before she can throw her punch. Then, you can hitch any punches you want on the back end of your jab. Today, try a right hook to the body.

◆ **Step + Straight Right + Left Hook + Right Uppercut + Left Hook:** The straight right works as a counter if you can get inside the left hook. Take a quick step up and to the left, and pivoting your right foot and powering through the hips, deliver your right directly between your opponent's chin and chest. Chances are, she won't have enough time to

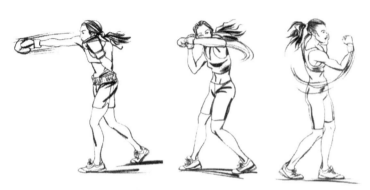

get the hook off, but, just in case, keep your chin tucked so your head remains protected by your right shoulder. You can followup your right with anything you can think of. Today, make it a 4-punch combination; add a left hook, a right uppercut, and another left hook.

◆ **Elbow Block (right) + 1 + 2:** The moment you read the left hook to the body—your opponent drops, and her elbow comes away from her ribs—prepare to block it with your right elbow. She'll spring back to snake position, and you'll be ready with your quickest 1-2 punch.

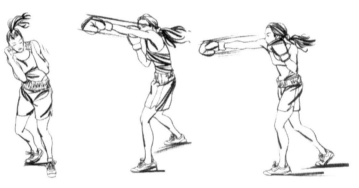

## 1 Minute: Rest

## 3 Minutes: Shadowboxing: Countering Right Hooks

Defending yourself against and countering the right hook to either the chin or body is very similar to defending yourself against the left hook for obvious reasons. Also, remember bobbing and weaving. It makes for particularly good defense against hooks, as you duck down and step to the same side as the hook. It'll open up an entire side of her body to you.

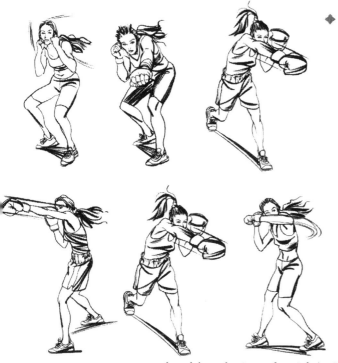

- **Duck + One-Two to the Body:** Drop down, keeping your back straight, to allow the hook to pass overhead. While you're in a squat position, counter with a jab to the body, followed by a straight right to the body.

- **Step + Jab + Straight Right to the Body + Left Hook:** As soon as you see your opponent's right elbow lift, take a step toward her and jab her hard in the chin before she can land her right hook. (Even if you're slow, keep your chin tucked so your face remains protected by your left shoulder during the jab.) Squat quickly for a straight right to the body—this will cover you if she's throwing a double hook—and finish with a left hook to her chin.

- **Elbow Block (left) + Right Overhand + Left Hook:** Intercept her right hook to your body with a braced left-elbow block, and as she stands up, answer her with a right overhand, followed by a quick left hook.

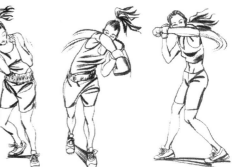

## 1 Minute: Rest

## 3 Minutes: Shadowboxing

Build your hand pacing and stamina with another 3-minute speed round. There are an infinite number of combinations to throw, but today you'll learn just three more. Go easy for the first 45 seconds of each minute and finish up with rapid-fire punches during the last 15 seconds. If your brain gets stuck and you can't think of which combination to deliver, just keep doing the same one until something new comes to you. You always want to have another combination on deck, even if it is the same one.

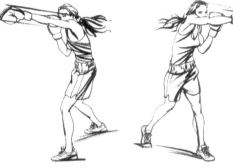

- **Jab + Right Cross + Jab:** Get back to basics with this combination, making sure your jab lands in exactly the same place each time.

- **Straight Right to the Body + Left Hook to the Body + Right Hook + Left Hook:** Work your way up your opponent's body with this combination. Work on clean pivots with every punch.

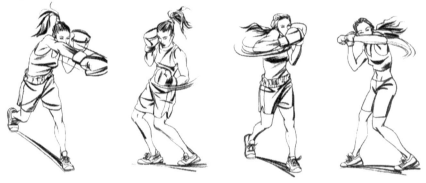

- **Jab + Right Uppercut + Straight Right:** If your opponent is tired and you're not, this is a great sequence. It's not the safest punch series to throw—the right side of your face may be open for a split second because your right

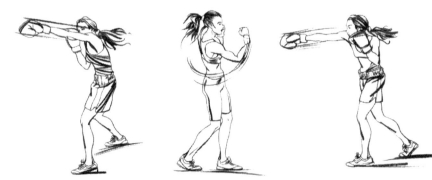

hand is doing all the work and not there to protect your chin. But if you do it quickly and are ready to duck or slip right to avoid counters, you'll be fine. Your opponent, however, won't be.

## 1 Minute: Rest

## 15 Minutes: Strength Training

You've already practiced these moves 1 times before, so eke out a few more reps of each today to keep them challenging. Again, rest for 30 seconds between sets, and to keep your heart rate elevated, rest only for 30 seconds, instead of your usual minute, between moves, too.

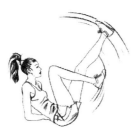

### Bicycle

*Do 3 sets of 75.*

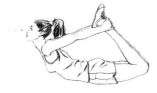

### Bow

*Do 1 set of 3 reps, holding the pose for 20 seconds and resting for 10 seconds between each rep.*

### Triangle Push-ups

*Do 3 sets of 8. Use your knees if need be.*

### Flutter Kicks

*Do 3 sets of 20.*

# Day Three: Countering Uppercuts
## THE OVERVIEW

Uppercuts are always thrown at close range, and like the hook, they can be read early. Many boxers, especially tired ones, advertise their uppercuts by pulling their fists down to their hips before firing. That's your window of opportunity. Since you never want to lean away from a punch, your best defense against an uppercut is your speed. Counter fast and hard.

# What You're Doing Today:
## WEEK THREE, DAY THREE

| | |
|---|---|
| 12 Minutes: | Jump Rope |
| | *3 Minutes @ Level 3–4* |
| | *1 Minute @ Level 5–6* |
| | *5 Minutes @ Level 7–8* |
| | *3 Minutes @ Level 3–4* |
| 1 Minute: | Rest |
| 3 Minutes: | Shadowboxing: Countering Right Uppercuts |
| | *Jab + Left Hook + Left Hook to the Body* |
| | *Jab + Left Hook + Straight Right + Right Hook* |
| | *Retreat + Triple Jab* |
| 1 Minute: | Rest |
| 3 Minutes: | Shadowboxing: Countering Left Uppercuts |
| | *Right Hook + Double Right Hook to the Body* |
| | *Straight Right + Left Hook + Straight Right + Left Hook* |
| | *Retreat + Jab + Jab to the Body + Right Cross* |

| | |
|---|---|
| 1 Minute: | Rest |
| 3 Minutes: | Shadowboxing |
| | *1 + 2 + 3 + 4 + Left Hook* |
| | *Jab + Right Uppercut + Left Hook + Straight Right + Left Hook* |
| | *Jab + Right Uppercut + Straight Right + Left Hook + Straight Right* |
| 15 Minutes: | Strength Training |
| | *Walking Lunges: 3 sets of 15* |
| | *Chest Push-Ups: 3 sets of 10* |
| | *Leg Raises: 3 sets of 15* |
| | *Supermans: 1 set of 3, holding for 20 seconds* |

# The Details

### 12 Minutes: Jump Rope

For nearly 3 weeks, you've been working on stretching your intense bouts of cardio out a bit longer every day. Today, after a 3-minute warm-up at level 3–4, ease into a level 5–6 for 1 minute. Once you've got your rhythm, then try to go for a full 5 minutes at level 7–8. Don't worry. You've already done 4 minutes at level 7–8 before, just not all at once. You can do it: By following this workout, you've built your lung capacity and your strength. Besides, a good trainer would never give a fighter more than she's ready for. You're ready for this. Cool down for 3 minutes at a level 3–4.

### 1 Minute: Rest

### 3 Minutes: Shadowboxing: Countering Right Uppercuts

The right uppercut is often the last punch of a series, delivered on the re-treat. Take advantage of the fact that your opponent's weight is tipping to her back foot, and knock her off balance with a hard, quick punch. Your other option is to simply move out of your opponent's range. The uppercut is a close-range punch. If you shuffle back (never lean back) so you're out of reach, you remove the punch entirely from the match.

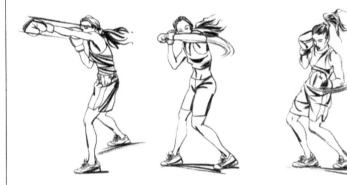

◆ **Jab + Left Hook + Left Hook to the Body:** Since she's dropped her right hand for the uppercut, the right side of her head is left unprotected.

◆ **Jab + Left Hook + Straight Right + Right Hook:** Lead with your left again, but this time finish with your right.

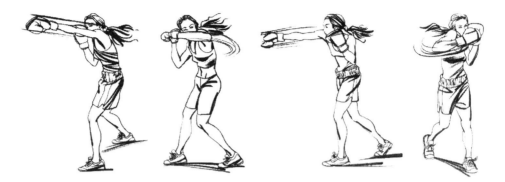

◆ **Retreat + Triple Jab:** Every move in this sequence is about making space for yourself to regroup. The jab is a long-range punch, which means you can still hit your opponent even though you're out of range for her uppercut.

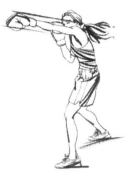

1 Minute: Rest

3 Minutes: Shadowboxing: Countering Left Uppercuts

When your opponent delivers a left uppercut, especially if she telegraphs the punch with an obvious wind-up, you've got an opening for some big right hands.

◆ **Right Hook + Double Right Hook to the Body:** As soon as you see her left fist drop, deliver a thumb-up right hook. Then, from a squatting position, punch her twice in the side with 2 right hooks to the body. Power the punches from your hips by pivoting your back foot.

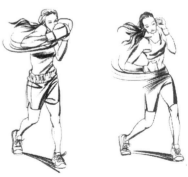

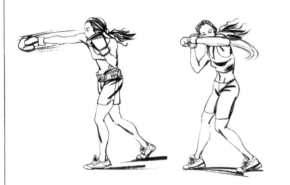

◆ **Straight Right + Left Hook + Straight Right + Left Hook:** If you're a power puncher, this is your dream combination. Just don't get so overzealous that you push your punches. Keep your weight balanced, so if you miss, you won't stumble.

◆ **Retreat + Jab + Jab to the Body + Right Cross:** A quick step back will make any uppercut meaningless. Answer with long-range punches: a jab, a jab to the body, and a lengthy right cross.

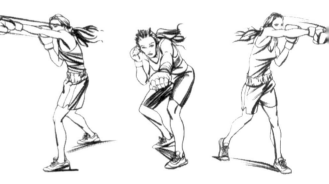

## 1 Minute: Rest

## 3 Minutes: Shadowboxing

This is the last speed drill of the week, so make it count. It's the same as the other two days: Go for 45 seconds at a relaxed pace, and then execute a flurry of punches for the last 15 seconds. Do not stop punching until you hit the minute mark. It's at the end of rounds, when boxers let their guards down, that matches turn. This round, try working on your first 5-punch combinations. If that's too much to remember, try practicing one combination for an entire minute before moving onto the next. Incorporate movement (circling, running the cross, and bobbing and weaving) to keep things real—and interesting.

◆ **1 + 2 + 3 + 4 + Left Hook:** You've already practiced this classic 4-punch combination—jab, straight right, left hook, and right uppercut. Top it off with a surprise left hook.

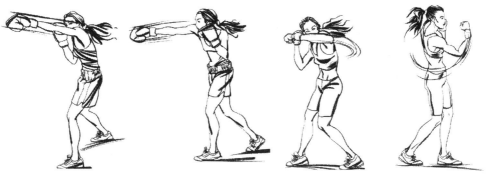

◆ **Jab + Right Uppercut + Left Hook + Straight Right + Left Hook:** This combination works just about every muscle in your body. Stay focused on your mental goals, so you can get through it.

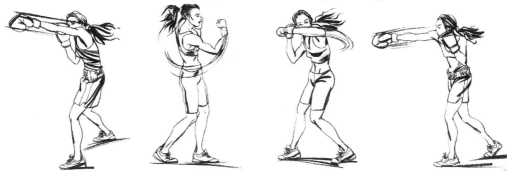

◆ **Jab + Right Uppercut + Straight Right + Left Hook + Straight Right:** If you're too tired to keep at it, try running the cross and delivering this combination at every end point. Watch your form. Tired fighters tend to get sloppy, but remember, technique, not power, wins matches.

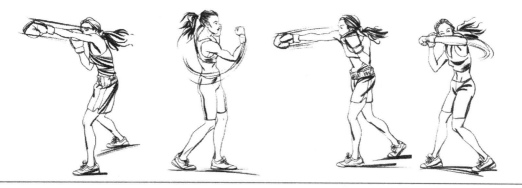

## 15 Minutes: Strength Training

Rest for 30 seconds between sets and moves today. For an added challenge, hold light weights in each hand during the walking lunges.

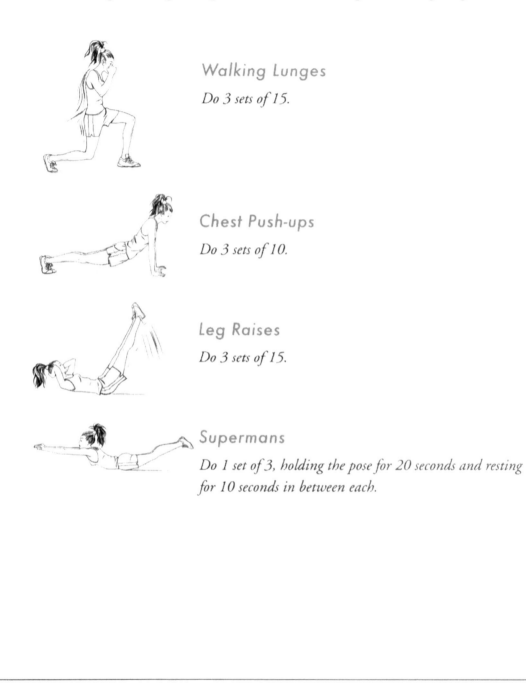

### Walking Lunges

*Do 3 sets of 15.*

### Chest Push-ups

*Do 3 sets of 10.*

### Leg Raises

*Do 3 sets of 15.*

### Supermans

*Do 1 set of 3, holding the pose for 20 seconds and resting for 10 seconds in between each.*

# Parting Shots

Now that you've learned to counterpunch and string together 5-punch combinations, you've proven that boxing moves are becoming natural to you, and you're getting fast on your feet. At Gleason's, we believe that listening to exactly what your trainer says is key. But there is room for a little improvisation. You're improving, getting stronger, and more confident, so, go ahead and have a little attitude, especially when counterpunching. It's now okay to add some of your own style. Show some finesse and creativity; you've earned it.

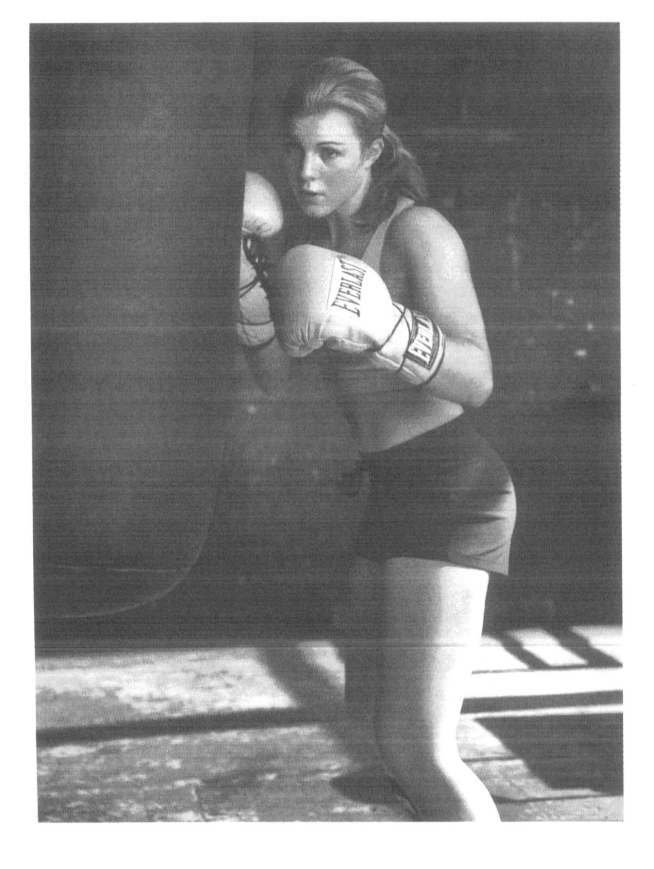

# 9

# Week Four:

## Become a Knockout

**Y**ou've come this far, and you've shown that both your body and mind have grown more powerful and fit. By the end of this week, you will look and feel stronger, fitter, faster, and leaner than you ever have before. You *will* have a boxer's body. Take what you've built and move to the next level. Prove you can go the distance, and push yourself even harder.

## Your Fighting Focus:

If you've done all your work up until now, then by the end of this week, you will be fully prepared to go into the ring to spar with another fighter—and win. You already know how to move, punch, and counterpunch. This week, you'll add two new skills to what you know. First, you'll learn to string several four-punch combinations together. The purpose of all the shadowboxing you've done in the past three weeks is to get your hands and body to move automatically, by reflex. If you stutter or have to stop to think about what you should do next, you'll be hit. You want to get into the habit of sliding from one combination to the next without thinking about it, so you can take full advantage of any openings you get in the ring. The second new skill you'll acquire this week is learning how to fight as a southpaw—or if you're already a southpaw, fighting orthodox, which means right-handed. Knowing how to fight from a different stance is sometimes all it takes to win a match. The simple switch can be enough to throw off your opponent by tripping up her defense. Consider it a secret weapon in your fighting arsenal.

## Your Fitness Focus:

All month you've been using intervals to build your endurance—resting and sprinting to accumulate as much high-intensity work as your body could handle in the shortest amount of time. As a result, your heart has become stronger. Your circulatory system has become better equipped to move blood and oxygen to the muscles faster. Your lungs have become more efficient, able to fill themselves with more air during each inhalation. Your muscles have adjusted to working so hard by becoming stronger. Now, it's time to reap the benefits.

This month, you'll move into high-intensity steady-state work or working harder with less rest. That means you'll burn more calories during your jump rope session than you did before because you now skip the rest periods. Through your shadowboxing, you'll continue to build your endurance. During round one, use your stamina and mental prowess to throw eight punches in a row over and over again. During round two, you'll switch your stances, forcing your muscles to work from different angles. The change forces your muscles to adapt quickly, rather than you relying on the same moves all the time. Performing new moves means new challenges for your muscles, which translates into more definition faster. You know what the third round brings: speed drills, as usual. This is where your endurance really kicks in. Finally, during your strength-training session, you'll continue to build on your repetitions.

# The Workouts: Week Four

## Day One: Putting it All Together
### THE OVERVIEW

While jumping rope—15 minutes today, up from last week's 12 minutes—and during the first 2 of the 3 rounds of shadowboxing, focus only on your rhythm, not your speed. The idea is to build your reflexes so that you can be more responsive in the ring. The punch combos you string together today all have one thing in common: They begin the same way but end differently. Practicing them this way will give you the skills you'll need to change up your attack, midpunch, without hesitation.

## What You're Going to Do Today:
### WEEK FOUR, DAY ONE

| | |
|---|---|
| 15 Minutes: | Jump Rope |
| | *3 Minutes @ Level 5–6* |
| | *6 Minutes @ Level 7–8* |
| | *4 Minutes @ Level 5–6* |
| | *2 Minutes @ Level 3–4* |
| 1 Minute: | Rest |
| 3 Minutes: | Shadowboxing |
| | *1 + 2 + 1 + 2 with 1 + 2 + Left Hook + Left Hook to the Body* |
| | *Triple Jab + Right Uppercut with Triple Jab + Left Hook to the Body* |

Jab + Left Hook + Right Uppercut + Left Upper
cut with Jab + Left Hook + Right Uppercut
+ Right Hook

| 1 Minute: | Rest |
|---|---|
| 3 Minutes: | Shadowboxing<br>*Run the Cross with 1 + 2s*<br>*Jab + Duck + 1 + 2*<br>*1 + 2 + 3* |
| 1 Minute: | Rest |
| 3 Minutes: | Shadowboxing<br>Jab + Right Uppercut + Left Hook + Straight<br>    Right + Left Hook<br>Jab + Right Uppercut + Straight Right +<br>    Left Hook + Straight Right<br>1 + 2 + 3 + 4 + Left Hook |
| 1 Minute: | Rest |
| 15 Minutes: | Strength Training<br>*Jump Squats: 3 sets of 15*<br>*Alligator Push-ups: 3 sets of 12*<br>*Side Scissors: 3 sets of 20*<br>*Twist Crunches: 3 sets of 20* |

# The Details

### 15 Minutes: Jump Rope

Begin today's warm-up at a slightly faster pace than usual; shoot for a level 5–6. After the 3-minute mark, kick it up to a full level 7–8 for 6 minutes. Recover with 4 minutes on a level 5–6, and cool down with another 3 minutes on level 3–4. If you want to spice things up, try jumping one-footed. Just remember to alternate your feet, so your calves, thighs, and butt get a balanced workout.

### 1 Minute: Rest

### 3 Minutes: Shadowboxing

Now that you've got many of the basic combinations down, practice two together *without* sacrificing your technique. Go slow at first so you get it right. Throwing a sloppy punch is far worse for you than not throwing a punch at all. The only person in the ring it'll slow down is you. Once you have the technique down, try varying your delivery: String all 8 punches together in one run. Deliver your first four, add a defensive maneuver, such as a duck or slip in between, and then finish with the last four. Try a few where you throw the second combination first. Keep moving.

◆ **1 + 2 + 1 + 2 with 1 + 2 + Left Hook + Left Hook to the Body:** The jab and straight right are lethal openers to any combination since they're so quick. You distract your opponent with the jab to set up your

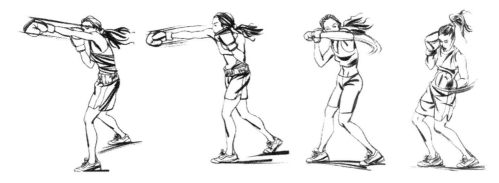

power punch. Always be prepared to continue your assault. If you need to be quick, try a second 1+2. If you have another beat of time or if your opponent drops her right fist, a couple of left hooks can really catch her off guard.

◆ **Triple Jab + Right Uppercut with Triple Jab + Left Hook to the Body:** Often times, you'll use the triple jab to create some space between you and your opponent. If she still manages to get close, be ready to deliver a hard short-range punch: either an uppercut or hook to the body.

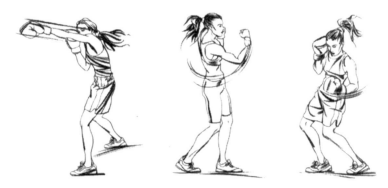

◆ **Jab + Left Hook + Right Uppercut + Left Uppercut with Jab + Left Hook + Right Uppercut + Right Hook:** You're only changing up 1 punch in these combinations; you'll swap the left uppercut for the right hook.

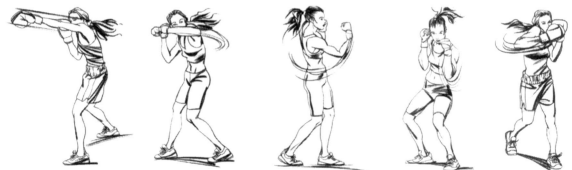

1 Minute: Rest

During your rest period, refresh your memory about the southpaw stance. Stand with your feet, shoulder-width apart, with your left foot about 18 inches *behind* your right, left toe pointed out at slightly wider than 45-degree angle. Your right toe should be pointing toward your opponent. Keep your weight centered and your belly button sucked in toward your spine. Raise both of your fists to your tucked chin. Your jab will come from your *right* hand. Your power punches will come from your *left*. When switching stances, there's the natural tendency to push your punches. Avoid this pitfall by pivoting on the balls of your feet and powering through your hips, not your shoulders.

## 3 Minutes: Shadowboxing

It's back to basics today for your first attempt at fighting southpaw. Get your stance right first. Then practice your movement. Finally, start throwing punches.

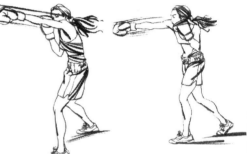

◆ **Run the Cross with 1 + 2s:** You're learning to move all over again. Remember to step forward first with your front (right) foot and then follow with your left (back) foot. When you're retreating, you'll step back first with your left (back) foot and follow it with your right (front) foot. Once you get the hang of the shuffling, try adding a 1+2 punch at the end point of your cross. Advance, 1+2. Retreat, 1+2. Right, 1+2. Left, 1+2. And so on. Remember, jab as if you're screwing your fist into your opponent. Don't push your punch. Don't lean. Don't cross your feet.

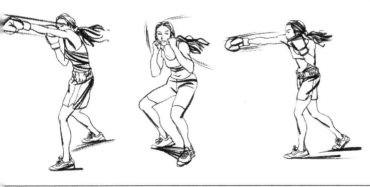

◆ **Jab + Duck + 1 + 2:** And don't forget your defense. Throw a jab to your opponent's chin with your right hand. Duck while keeping your back straight and your eyes on her; then take a step toward your opponent and throw a 1+2—jab with your right hand and follow with your left hand.

◆ **1 + 2 + 3:** Jab with your right hand, follow it with a straight left to the chin, and finish with a right hook. Remember to hold your hand as if you're holding a beer mug when you do the right hook. This combination can be especially effective, since your right arm is probably the more powerful of the 2. You may be able to hit harder and faster with it.

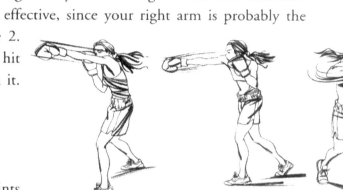

## 1 Minute: Rest

## 3 Minutes: Shadowboxing

The way you score points in a real match is by throwing slick combinations of punches. Tossing a lot of different punches into the mix throws off your opponent. Therefore, during this round, do speed drills. Switch back to your usual stance. If you're right handed, go back to the orthodox stance; if you're a lefty, return to the southpaw stance. Now alternate 30 seconds of punching at a moderate pace with a full 30 seconds at a fast pace. You'll try some 5-punch combinations today, listed below. They'll give your body—and your brain—a workout. During the intense intervals, punch, move, and duck. Just do it fast. Your pace should be quick enough so that your heart is pounding.

◆ **Jab + Right Uppercut + Left Hook + Straight Right + Left Hook:** Get the rhythm down: left, right, left, right, left. Go as fast as you can without sacrificing your form. For some people that'll be a lot slower

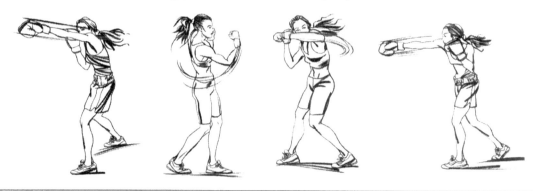

than during the 2-and 3-punch combinations. Others will be able to pull this off without a second thought. If you lose your place, just create your own sequence. You need to learn to think on your feet.

◆ **Jab + Right Uppercut + Straight Right + Left Hook + Straight Right:** Your hooks and rights simply switch position in this combination.

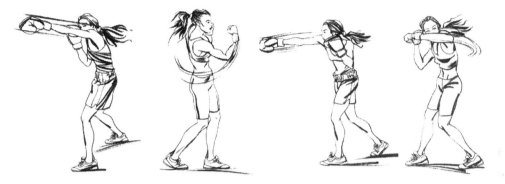

◆ **1 + 2 + 3 + 4 + Left Hook:** Throw a jab, straight right, left hook, and right uppercut, and finish off with a left hook. If you can pull this off in a match, you'll be wearing the Golden Gloves in no time.

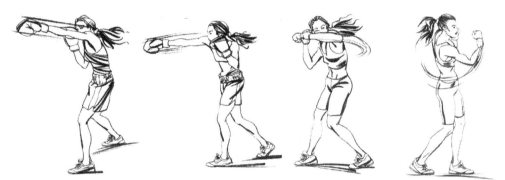

## 1 Minute: Rest

## 15 Minutes: Strength Training

Take the same amount of rest today as you did last week: 30 seconds between sets and 30 seconds between moves. It'll keep your heart rate elevated, which will burn more calories and increase your endurance.

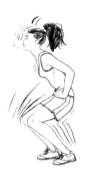

## Jump Squats

*Do 3 sets of 15.*

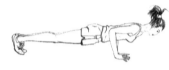

## Alligator Push-ups

*Do 3 sets of 12. Drop to your knees, if you need to.*

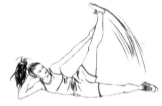

## Side Scissors

*Do 3 sets of 20.*

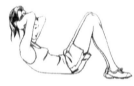

## Twist Crunches

*Do 3 sets of 20.*

# Day Two: Get Your Head Together
## THE OVERVIEW

The training wheels (so to speak) come off today. After 15 minutes of jumping rope—not longer, just a little harder—a round's worth of throwing more 4-punch combinations in rapid succession, and a round's worth of fighting southpaw, you're going to do your own round of freestyle fighting. That is, it's up to you to figure out which combinations you want to throw when. (*Psst.* This is the part where you get to show off a little bit.)

# What You're Going to Do Today:
## WEEK FOUR, DAY TWO

| | |
|---|---|
| 15 Minutes: | Jump Rope |
| | *4 Minutes @ Level 5–6* |
| | *7 Minutes @ Level 7–8* |
| | *4 Minutes @ Level 5–6* |
| 1 Minute: | Rest |
| 3 Minutes: | Shadowboxing |
| | *Jab + Straight Right + Jab to the Body + Straight Right to the Body with Straight Right to the Body + Left Uppercut + Right Uppercut + Jab* |
| | *Left Hook to the Body + Right Hook to the Body + Left Hook + Right Hook with Left Hook + Right Hook + Left Hook to the Body + Right Hook to the Body* |

*Straight Right to the Body + Right Hook to the Body + Right Hook + Right Cross with Jab + Left Hook + Left Hook to the Body + Jab to the Body*

| | |
|---|---|
| 1 Minute: | Rest |
| 3 Minutes: | Shadowboxing |

*Jab + Left Hook to the Body*
*Jab + Jab to the Body + Right Hook*
*Jab + Right Uppercut + Left Hook*

| | |
|---|---|
| 1 Minute: | Rest |
| 3 Minutes: | Shadowboxing |

*Freestyle*

| | |
|---|---|
| 1 Minute: | Rest |
| 15 Minutes: | Strength Training |

*Bicycle: 2 sets of 100*
*Bow: 1 set of 3, 25-second holds*
*Triangle Push-ups: 2 sets of 15*
*Flutter Kicks: 3 sets of 25*

# The Details

## 12 Minutes: Jump Rope

Push yourself hard right now. It will pay off: You're melting off about 141 calories in these first 12 minutes of your workout (more if you weigh more than 135 pounds). Warm up for 3 minutes at a level 5–6, then go all out for a full 2 rounds, or 6 minutes, at a level 7–8. Recover during your final 3-minute round by cruising at level 5–6.

## 1 Minute: Rest

## 3 Minutes: Shadowboxing

While it may be rare that you'd actually get to throw any of these particular eight punches in a row in the ring, give them a try today. They'll help you fine tune your placement, which may tend to get a little wild depending on the amount of pressure you're under or if you're feeling a little tired.

◆ **Jab + Straight Right + Jab to the Body + Straight Right to the Body with Straight Right to the Body + Left Uppercut + Right Uppercut + Jab:** The first combination runs down the center of your opponent's body. The second combination runs up it. Move sharply back into snake position between the 2 combinations, and be sure to keep your back straight when you squat. See if you can target the same landing point with equal precision on your rights and lefts.

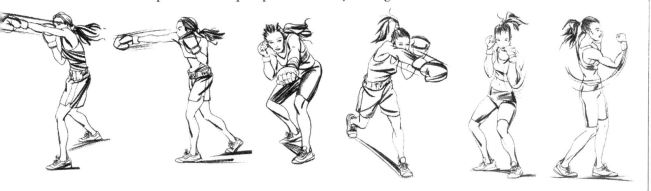

◆ **Left Hook to the Body + Right Hook to the Body + Left Hook + Right Hook with Left Hook + Right Hook + Left Hook to the Body + Right Hook to the Body:** Work your way up and down the sides of your opponent—from the ribs to the chin—with these hooks. Remember to pivot your front foot on the left hook and your back foot on the right hook to summon power from your hips.

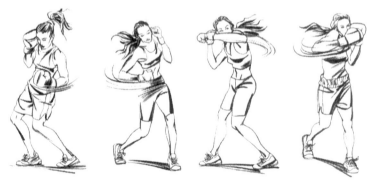

◆ **Straight Right to the Body + Right Hook to the Body + Right Hook + Right Cross with Jab + Left Hook + Left Hook to the Body + Jab to the Body:** Do a 1-handed assault on the way up and a 1-handed assault on the way down. Imagine punching a C-shape, backward and forward, into your opponent.

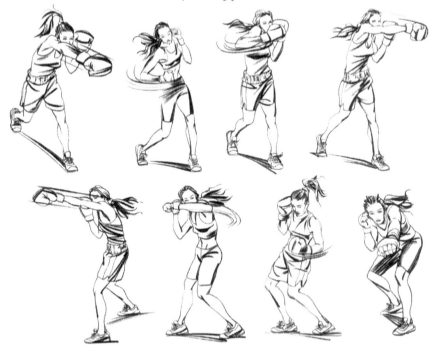

## 1 Minute: Rest

## 3 Minutes: Shadowboxing

Try fighting as a southpaw again during this round and keep on practicing the basics until throwing a jab with your right hand—screwing it out with a snap—feels as natural as it does with your left.

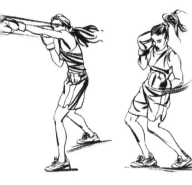

◆ **Jab + Left Hook to the Body:** After throwing the jab, squat down and pivot your back foot as you swing through your hips to deliver your left hook to the body. Since you've switched stances, remember that your left forearm should be parallel to the floor and your left fist should be positioned with your thumb up and your palm facing you.

◆ **Jab + Jab to the Body + Right Hook:** This is a right-handed attack. On the hook, your right fist should be palm down, with your thumb facing you.

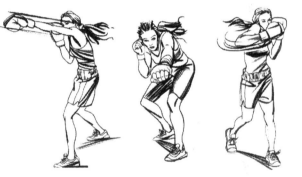

◆ **Jab + Right Uppercut + Left Hook:** Keep your left hand up to protect your chin during the first 2 punches and try not to telegraph your uppercut by dramatically pulling your right fist low. During the hook, keep your thumb up and your palm facing you.

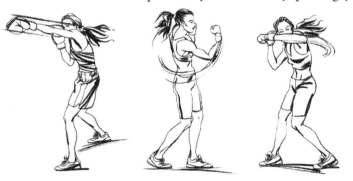

## 1 Minute: Rest

## 3 Minutes: Shadowboxing: Freestyle

By now you've probably practiced more combinations than you'd ever have a chance to actually use in a match. So freestyle during this round by putting different combinations together. Bob, weave, slip, duck, and circle. Throw single punches. Do whatever comes to you. Your goal today is to visualize each 3-minute bout during the rest period. Know what you're going to throw two combinations ahead of the one you're throwing and continue your speed work by ending each minute with ten to 30 seconds of fast fighting.

## 1 Minute: Rest

## 15 Minutes: Strength Training

Rest for 30 seconds between sets and moves today.

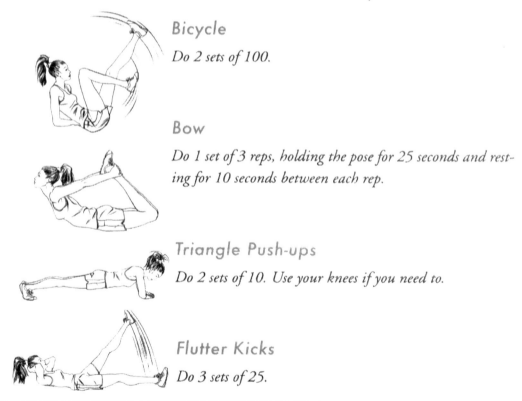

### Bicycle
*Do 2 sets of 100.*

### Bow
*Do 1 set of 3 reps, holding the pose for 25 seconds and resting for 10 seconds between each rep.*

### Triangle Push-ups
*Do 2 sets of 10. Use your knees if you need to.*

### Flutter Kicks
*Do 3 sets of 25.*

# Day Three: Be Your Own Champion
## THE OVERVIEW

This is the last official day of the program, so make it really count. After this, you can freestyle by keeping up your jumping rope intensity and mixing and matching the exercises and shadowboxing combinations that you enjoy. As you enter the final stretch, maintain a high intensity throughout the entire workout. We want you to push yourself all the way to end. Ahead, you've got 15 minutes of jumping rope, a round of double combinations, a round of southpaw basics, and another round of freestyling. Finish off with your strength moves and then go celebrate. You're fit, focused, and ready to spar.

# What You're Going to Do Today:
## WEEK FOUR, DAY THREE

| | |
|---|---|
| 15 Minutes: | Jump Rope |
| | *3 Minutes @ Level 5–6* |
| | *9 Minutes @ Level 7–8* |
| | *3 Minutes @ Level 3–4* |
| 1 Minute: | Rest |
| 3 Minutes: | Shadowboxing |
| | *Jab + Right Uppercut + Left Hook to the Body + Left Hook with Straight Right to the Body + Straight Right + Left Hook to the Body + Left Hook* |
| | *Jab + Left Uppercut + Right Hook + Right Hook with Jab to the Body Straight Right to the Body + Right Hook + Right Hook* |

*Jab + Straight Right + Jab + Jab with Jab +*
*Right Hook to the Body + Jab + Jab*

| | |
|---|---|
| 1 Minute: | Rest |
| 3 Minutes: | Shadowboxing: Southpaw<br>*Jab + Straight Left + Right Hook to the Body +*<br>*Left Hook to the Body Jab + Left Uppercut*<br>*+ Right Hook + Right Hook Jab + Left*<br>*Uppercut + Right Uppercut + Left Hook* |
| 1 Minute: | Rest |
| 3 Minutes: | Shadowboxing<br>*Freestyle* |
| 1 Minute: | Rest |
| 15 Minutes: | Strength Training<br>*Walking Lunges: 2 sets of 25*<br>*Chest Push-ups: 3 sets of 12*<br>*Leg Raises: 2 sets of 25*<br>*Supermans: 1 set of 2, holding for 30 seconds* |

# The Details

## 12 Minutes: Jump Rope

Stretch it out; you can do it. This is the same as last time: Warm up for a 3-minute round at a level 5–6. Then go wild for longer than you've ever gone—7 minutes at a level 7–8. Remember, working out at a level 7–8 of intensity doesn't necessarily mean you're going to maintain the same exact speed through the 7 minutes. At the beginning, you may rate 1 speed that intense. At the end, you may need to go faster or slower to maintain the same intensity level, depending on how you feel. Cool down for 3 minutes at a nice and easy level 3–4. But stamina is critical, so don't stop. You aren't finished yet. Nobody's getting knocked out. You've got to go the distance.

## 1 Minute: Rest

## 3 Minutes: Shadowboxing

Earlier in the week, you worked on punches that begin the same but end differently. Today, you're going to work on putting two combinations together that begin differently but end the same.

◆ **Jab + Right Uppercut + Left Hook to the Body + Left Hook with Straight Right to the Body + Straight Right + Left Hook to the Body + Left Hook:** Make your body shots count by really squatting down, until your thighs are almost parallel to the ground.

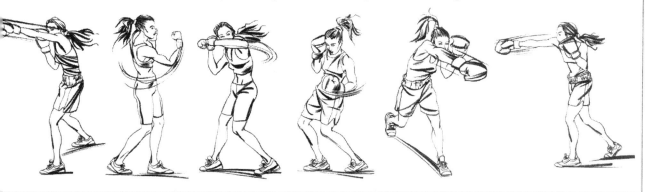

◆ **Jab + Left Uppercut + Right Hook + Right Hook with Jab to the Body + Straight Right to the Body + Right Hook + Right Hook:** Finishing off with a double hook is great punishment for those fighters who drop their hands or untuck their chin. As you begin the second combination, step into it as you deliver the jab to the body.

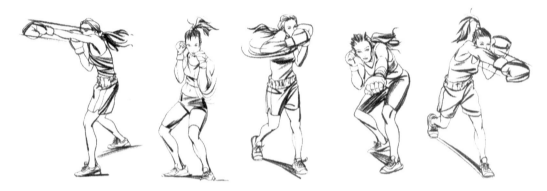

◆ **Jab + Straight Right + Jab + Jab with Jab + Right Hook to the Body + Jab + Jab:** The purpose of these jabs is to keep your opponent off balance and distracted while you set up for more punches.

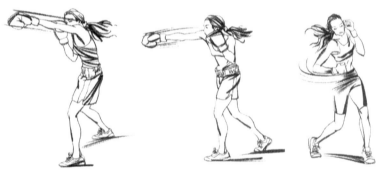

## 1 Minute: Rest

## 3 Minutes: Shadowboxing: Southpaw

Switch to your southpaw stance again and try a few of the combinations today. You've already practiced these in your orthodox stance. See how they feel when you're fighting lefty.

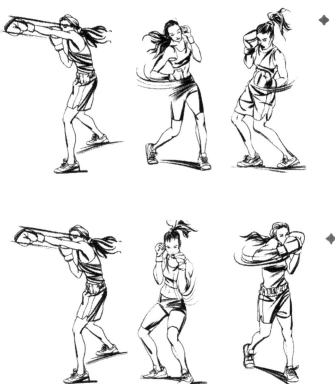

◆ **Jab + Straight Left + Right Hook to the Body + Left Hook to the Body:** Jab with your right hand, then throw a left. Your palm should be facing you on both hooks to the body; only your right hook should move in *and* up, and your left hook should move parallel to the ground.

◆ **Jab + Left Uppercut + Right Hook + Right Hook:** Be sure to punch up through to the ceiling on your uppercut. On both right hooks to the chin, your palm should be facing down.

◆ **Jab + Left Uppercut + Right Uppercut + Left Hook:** This is a particularly effective combination when you're within close range to your opponent. Keep your chin tucked and your weight evenly balanced on both feet. Never lean back.

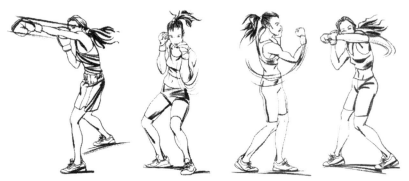

1 Minute: Rest

## 3 Minutes: Shadowboxing: Freestyle

Your last goal with freestyle shadowboxing was to know which punches you planned to throw two combinations ahead of time. Today, see if you can plan even further ahead. Your goal this round is absolutely no hesitation. For the last 20 to 30 seconds of each minute, try speeding up your hands to throw 2, 3, and even 4 combinations in a row.

## 15 Minutes: Strength Training

This is your final round of strength training, so really push yourself. As usual, rest for 30 seconds between sets and moves.

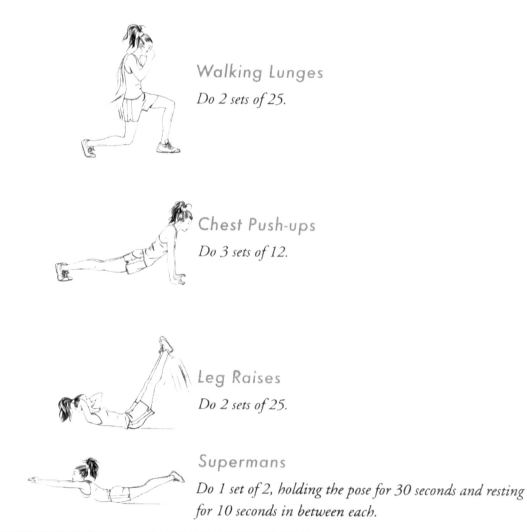

### Walking Lunges
*Do 2 sets of 25.*

### Chest Push-ups
*Do 3 sets of 12.*

### Leg Raises
*Do 2 sets of 25.*

### Supermans
*Do 1 set of 2, holding the pose for 30 seconds and resting for 10 seconds in between each.*

# Parting Shots

You did it. You now have what it takes to go into the ring. You don't have to, but you could. You've learned how to punch and counterpunch, how to move, how to defend yourself, and how to throw combinations. Your muscles are strong, and your lungs have stopped burning. You've honed your focus, reflexes, and concentration. Most of all, you've proven that you've got heart. Don't quit now: Feel free to continue the Gleason's workout by mixing, matching, and repeating what you've been taught. Or, take the next step: Get yourself a trainer and go into the ring.

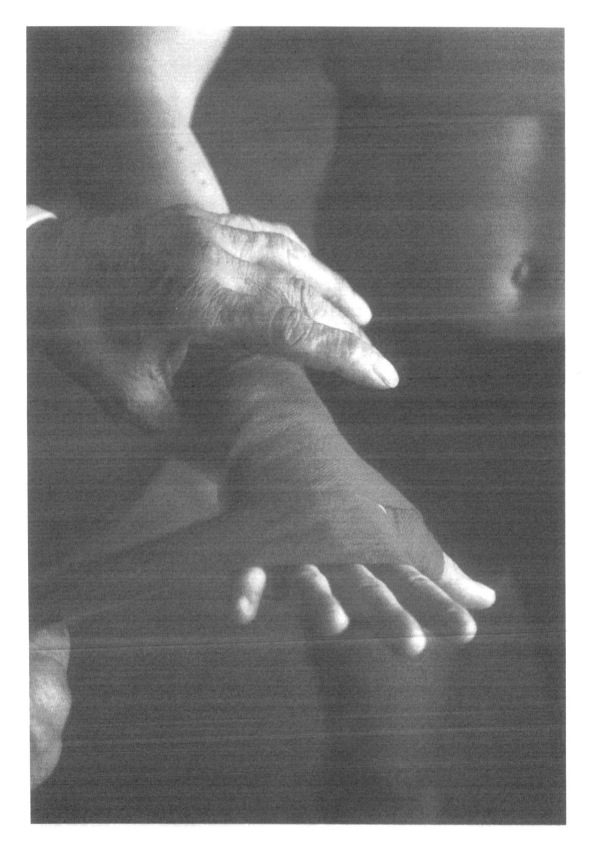

# 10
# The Next Level:
## Advancing Your Skills in the Gym

**C**ongratulations on continuing your boxing training! You may be like so many people who come into Gleason's, and the first thing they say is, "I just want to learn to box for fitness, but I don't want to ever *hit* anyone." But after several weeks of our workouts, boxing revs up their adrenaline, and they've caught the bug, changed their minds, and are antsy to step into the ring. Boxing is an exciting and addictive sport, and now that you're strong and fit and have some basic boxing skills under your belt, you may want to put yourself to the test and go for the real thing. Plus, the power, emotion, and confidence boxing inspires provides even more incentive to try your hand at fighting.

If so, you'll need some pointers on getting started. Here's a quick rundown of some of the major pieces of equipment you'll find in a boxing gym, along with some instructions for how to use them. While you can continue this workout on your own at home, you may want to take your skills to the next level and get competitive. Find a gym in your area, and hire yourself a trainer.

# How to Use The Heavy Bag

You don't pummel a 50- to 150-pound bag hanging from the ceiling to become more powerful. (That's what all those push-ups are for.) The purpose of training on a heavy bag is to learn how to land your punches in the right place in the right way. You use the bag to master your form and accuracy. It's also a great way to take out your aggression when you're having a bad day. It feels good. Here are three simple drills to try on the heavy bag.

**Drill One:** Circle the bag, practicing your jabs and 1+2. If the bag starts swinging when you're hitting it, you're pushing your punches.

**Drill Two:** Add the body shot into your heavy bag routine. Practice your 1+2-left hook to the body, left hook to the body, right hook to the body, and any other combinations you can think of that involve body shots. Keep circling. Don't let your eyes drop.

**Drill Three:** Put your punches together now. Go for a 1+2+3, then a right-left-right-left, then a few jabs to set up more body shots. Get used to the feeling of impact and landing your punches exactly where you're aiming. Your precision will be vital if you move into the ring and begin aiming for your opponent, who will be a lot faster than the bag.

## Heavy Bag Do's and Don'ts

1. Don't try and kill the bag. You want to land punches, not annihilate the equipment. Remember the basics.
2. Do look at the bag as you're punching. Too may people cock their arms back, and pull their heads up hoping to deliver a knockout punch. Instead stay in snake position and go for finesse, not force.
3. Don't stand in one place and hit the bag. Stay on the balls of your feet and move around the bag as you would in the ring.

# How to Use The Speed Bag

If you're slow getting off punches, the speed bag will become your new best friend. It'll improve your reflexes, give you faster fists, and improve your hand-eye coordination. But until you learn how to use it properly, take it slow. Here's what to do: Adjust the bag so it's at just higher than eye level, and stand in front of it in snake position. Don't move around the bag; stay in one place. Raise your right fist, as if you were going to deliver a right hook, only turn your fist so your palm is facing downward. Strike the bag once (and gently) with the outside of your right hand. Once it hits the backboard, strike it again. When you find your rhythm, add your left hand into the mix, holding it in standard left hook position (palm facing down).

**Drill One:** Alternate your hands in a circular motion: right, left, right, left.

**Drill Two:** Double up on your hands—right, right, left, left—and increase your speed. If you miss, just let the bag swing through and catch it again on its way toward you.

**Drill Three:** Practice combinations. Once you get your left-right-left rhythm, throw in an uppercut or a hook. You'll need quick reflexes and a good sense of timing to catch the bag in the proper position. If you miss, try to keep your balance. Recovery is an important lesson to learn in boxing.

## Speed Bag Do's and Don'ts

1. Don't try and break the bag to pieces. Remember the goal is to improve your reflexes and speed, not power.
2. Do start out slowly. It's okay to take it slow on a speed bag. If you go too fast, you'll never get the hang of it.
3. Do stop and start over if you lose control of the bag. Otherwise, you won't be able to land a solid punch.
4. Don't stand to the side of the bag. Face it head on.

# How to Use The Double End Bag

The double end bag is essentially a small punching ball tied with an elastic cord to the ceiling and floor. It's the closest you'll get to fighting a person without actually getting in the ring. Fighters call this "the crazy bag" because when you go after it, it comes back for you. That movement is why it's such a great tool for working on your slipping and circling. It'll also help you sharpen your punches. Try to hit fast, not hard. The best drill you can do with the double end bag is to jab and circle and jab and slip.

**Drill One:** Try and land a quick, 3-or 4-punch combination: left-right-left-right.

**Drill Two:** Do it again with a different combination: jab-right uppercut-left hook.

## Double End Bag Do's and Don'ts
1. Do hit the bag with your knuckles, not the side of your fist.
2. Don't try and hit the bag too hard.

# How to Use The Slipping Bag

The slipping bag looks almost like a speed bag, but it's heavier and swings from the ceiling on a chain. You do one thing with it: slip it while it swings.

## How to Slip
1. Begin in snake stance.
2. Take a step and bend your knees.
3. Turn your body so that you slip to the left of the bag.
4. Return to snake position.
5. Take a step and bend your knees.
6. Turn your body so that you slip to the right. Repeat for at least 3 minutes.

## Slipping Bag Do's and Don'ts

1. Don't drop your head to avoid the bag. Bend your knees.
2. Do move around. Step rather than just stand and bend your knees.

## ★ WHAT'S YOUR WEIGHT CLASS? ★

Step on the scale, and then check this chart to see what professional weight class you'd fall into if you were fighting in Gleason's home state of New York.

| Pounds | Class |
| --- | --- |
| 112 | Flyweight |
| 115 | Junior Bantamweight |
| 118 | Bantamweight |
| 122 | Junior Featherweight |
| 126 | Featherweight |
| 130 | Junior Lightweight |
| 135 | Lightweight |
| 140 | Junior Welterweight |
| 147 | Welterweight |
| 154 | Junior Middleweight |
| 160 | Middleweight |
| 168 | Super Middleweight |
| 175 | Light Heavyweight |
| 190 | Cruiserweight |
| Over 190 | Heavyweight |

## ★ GET EQUIPPED ★

If you're just going to train on the bags, all you need are hand wraps and gloves. If you're going to spar, you'll need protective headgear, a mouth guard, a groin protector, and a chest guard, too.

# Hand Wraps

A wrap is just a long piece of cotton cloth, about 2 inches wide, which boxers wind around their hands to support their joints, thumbs, knuckles, and wrists, from impact injuries. It generally has a cloth loop on one end and Velcro closures on the other. There are three types of wraps: short ones (150 inches), long ones (180 inches), and long ones with elastic. At Gleason's, our wrap of choice is the 180-inch elasticized long wrap ($1.79–$4.99). Gyms and sporting goods stores sell wrap, or try the Everlast website (www.everlast.com). The extra length equals extra protection, since you can wrap it around not only your knuckles and wrist, but also between your fingers. And the elasticity helps it form to your hand snugly. As far as the actual wrapping goes, there's no one right way to do it. We have seventy-seven other trainers working at Gleason's, and every one of them wraps their fighters' hands differently.

# Gloves

Boxing gloves come in different weights and different tie-up styles ($34.99–$89.99). You can buy gloves at boxing gyms, sporting goods stores, or on the website www.everlast.com. Choose your gloves based on what you plan to do in them.

Choose your style. If you're working out alone, go for the gloves with Velcro closures. You'll be able to get them on and off without any help. If you're working out in a gym or with a trainer, go for the lace-up gloves. They give your wrist more support and protection; you just need someone to tie them for you.

Now, figure out the weight. Gloves come in even-numbered weights, ranging from eight ounces up to twenty ounces. Choosing the weight of your gloves depends on what activities you plan to do in them. To shadowbox or hit bags, choose an eight-, ten-, or twelve-ounce glove. While the weight should have no bearing on your punch technique, it'll obviously add to the strenuousness of your workout. Generally, the heavier the glove on your hand, the faster you'll build muscle tone. For sparring, at Gleason's we require everyone under 160 pounds to wear fourteen-ounce gloves or heavier, and everyone over 160 pounds to wear sixteen-ounce gloves or heavier. A heavier glove eases impact by offering more padding and protection. It's the light gloves that do the most damage.

## ★ WRAP IT UP ★

### *How to Wrap Your Hands*

**Here is the easiest way to wrap. You may recognize this technique if you've ever sprained your wrist.**

1. Spread your fingers wide, with the palm side down.
2. Put your thumb through the loop at the end of the wrap.
3. Wrap around your wrist 3 or 4 times.
4. Stretch the wrap to the lower knuckle of your pinky and across the palm of your hand. The wrap should be snug, not tight.
5. Wrap across all of your knuckles and wrap around the back of your hand to your palm. Do this about 3 or 4 times as well.
6. Stretch the wrap diagonally across the back of your hand, around the front of your wrist, and around the knuckle of your thumb.
7. Wrap around your thumb and stretch it across the back of your hand.
8. Wrap across and around your thumb again, ending up on the front of your wrist.
9. Wrap around your wrist and diagonally across the back of your hand.
10. Wrap across your palm, around to the back of your wrist. Do this until you use up the wrap.
11. Secure with Velcro closure.

*(From www.everlast.com)*

## Mouthguards

Boil-and-bite mouthpieces not only help protect your teeth from getting knocked out and your lips from getting cut, but they also help keep your lower jaw stationary ($1.99–$25.99) They work this way: You boil the mouthpiece in hot water, let it cool slightly, and then stick it in your mouth and bite down. Once it cools, it adjusts to your mouth. If you get hit on the chin, your jaw won't knock into your skull and give you a concussion.

**Never step into the ring without a mouthguard.**

## Headgear

Boxing headgear is a foam helmet, which buckles under your chin and protects your head, cheeks, ears, and depending on the model, your nose ($29.99–$99.99). It'll also help protect your sparring partner's hands from your hard head. Get one snug enough so that it doesn't feel lose on your head, but not uncomfortably tight. We had one fighter come into Gleason's, and she was so worried about protecting her head that she bought the biggest headgear she could find. Needless to say, it only served to make her head a bigger target. She came in the next day with headgear that fit, and she fared much better in the ring.

## Groin Protector

Even women need the extra padding in case you get hit below the belt. Groin protectors, basically foam shorts with no behind, also serve to absorb blunt impact on many of your major organs. Most just lace up or hook in the back ($44.99–$99.99). You can buy them in boxing gyms, sporting goods stores, or on the website www.everlast.com

## Chest Protector

Here's your Madonna moment. A hit to the chest hurts, so at Gleason's we recommend that all women wear a chest protector. You can either buy specially-designed plastic cups to fit inside your sports bra, or you can go whole hog and get a foam pad to wear over your clothes ($29.99–$44.99). You can find them where other boxing products are sold.

### ★ WHICH BRAND IS BEST? ★

There are plenty of brands of boxing equipment, and a lot of them are really good, but at Gleason's, we only sell Everlast gear. That's because Gleason's is the official testing ground for all Everlast products. They develop equipment, and our fighters test it and give feedback. Then Everlast improves the gear until it meets Gleason's standards, so we know it's good stuff. You can order it from us at www.gleasonsgym.net, or you can get it directly from Everlast at www.everlastboxing.com.

### ★ HOW TO FIND A TRAINER ★

*Find someone who can communicate and listen.*

Because boxing is a sport that is based on survival—hitting and being hit—fear, anxiety, and self-doubt hang in the air, especially as a fight approaches. For high-level boxers in particular, the trainer serves not only as teacher and coach, but also as psychologist and cheerleader. When the stakes are high, a fighter may feel that the trainer is—literally—the only person really in her corner.

Finding a trainer that you trust and respect is key. There's no official licensing process for boxing trainers, though reputable gyms require some certification. It's important to be able to figure out if they know their stuff. Here are a few tips.

- Ask about experience. Try to get someone who's trained professional or amateur fighters, not just fitness fighters. If trainers have been around competition, chances are better that she knows her stuff.

- Watch. Go to your boxing gym and watch the trainers in action. Are they particular about technique? (If not, they're not worth your money.) Do they command respect from their fighters? Do they treat their fighters with respect? Are they focused on their fighters—or only half-paying attention?

- Listen. Your trainer should not only be able to communicate effectively with you, but also motivate you when you're feeling slow.

- Don't be afraid to shop around. Just because you hire someone for an hour, it doesn't mean he or she must be your trainer for life. It's ok to keep trying different trainers until you find one you click with. Good trainers understand this and won't take offense.

- Negotiate. We have seventy-eight trainers working at Gleason's, and we're all independent contractors. Most of us charge about $25 an hour for training, but most of us are also willing to make a deal. If you meet a trainer you like and really click with, but he or she is too expensive, don't be afraid to ask him or her about working out a deal.

# Parting Shots

We hope you've enjoyed our workout. You probably know by now that although boxing is best known for it's blood, sweat, and brutality, when done correctly and consistently, it's more about agility, finesse, and grace. As much as you've benefited physically from our workout with your leaner, stronger body, and increased levels of cardiovascular fitness, we also know that you've grown happier and more confident in all areas of your life. We hope we've taught you to focus your mind and listen to your body. Most of all, we hope we've treated you to not only the exhilaration of being an athlete and pushing beyond your limits, but also the joy and thrill of being a finer person.

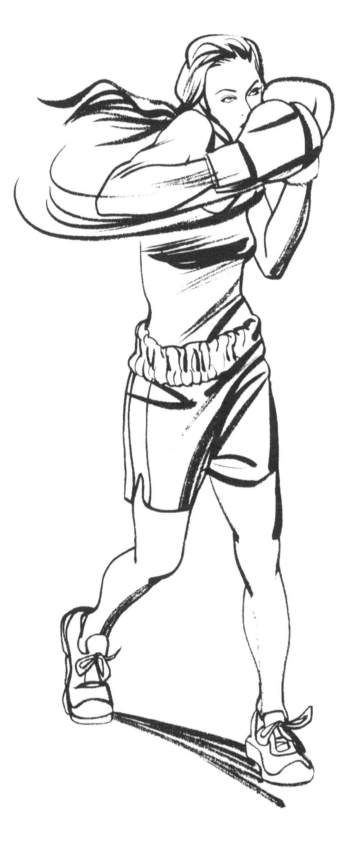

# Acknowledgments

We would like to acknowledge Robert "Bobby Gleason" Gagliardi, the original owener of Gleason's Gym, and Ira Becker, who took over the gym and invited us into the Gleason family. There wouldn't be a Gleason's without all of the trainers who have worked here throughout the years. Thank you for being the best at what you do. We are indebted to the success of the women's boxing movement and the numerous women's boxing champions who've dominated the New York City Golden Gloves. All of the women who train at Gleason's are champions to us, and we would especially like to thank those who participated in the photo shoot for this book: Christina Beckles, Angela Querol, Lawson Harris, Alexis Asher, Amy Bridges, Maureen Shea, Kathleen Hahn, and Ronica Jeffrey. Special thanks to Hilary Swank for supporting Gleason's Gym and this project.

We would like to thank our agent, Barbara Lowenstein. Thanks to Linda Villarosa and Erin Breid, who brought our expertise and our techniques to the page. David Lee at The Studio NYC captured movement and power in his illustrations. And Frank Veronsky captured the soul of Gleason's in his photographs. We would like to thank the entire team at Simon & Schuster, especially our editor, Nancy Hancock, Sarah Peach, and Jessica Napp. This book would not be what it is without each of your hard work and dedication.

I, Hector, would like to thank my mother, Gavina Ortega, for bringing me into this world.

I, Bruce, would like to thank my father Ed Silverglade, who got me started in boxing, and my wife, JoEllen VanOuwerkerk, an outstanding female boxer and my total support.

# About the Authors

**H**ector Roca was born on March 29, 1940 in Panama City.

Roca is well-known for the aspect of his training called "Learning the Power." He sees too many boxers trying to throw bombs and instead pushing their punches with far less power. Through detailed work on fundamentals and focusing on proper technique, Hector is gifted at maximizing his boxer's power.

Roca has been at Gleason's Gym longer than any other trainer.

*Boxing Digest* rated Roca the number one Spanish-speaking trainer in the world. He has worked with twelve world champions, including Arturo Gatti, Iran Barkley, and Buddy McGirt. His most famous boxer was Academy Award–winner Hilary Swank.

Hector currently resides in Brooklyn, New York.

**B**ruce Silverglade is president, owner, and operator of Gleason's Gym, Inc. The Silverglade name has been associated with boxing for more than seventy years. Bruce's father, Edward, was one of the founders of the

PAL. He also worked for the National Olympic Committee and was the team manager for the 1980 and 1984 U.S. Olympic teams.

In 1976, Bruce found himself in the middle of a divorce and sought refuge in boxing. While one marriage ended, another one was just beginning. Silverglade caught the boxing bug and quit his job of sixteen years with Sears Roebuck and Company. He began refereeing and judging amateur bouts, but because he liked "all" fighters, he quickly learned that he could not be an impartial official. That's when he turned to the administrative side of the sport.

From 1980 to 1985, Silverglade held some of the most prominent positions in amateur boxing. He was president of the Metropolitan Amateur Boxing Federation, a chairman of the National Junior Olympic Committee, and a member of the National Selection Committee.

By the mid-eighties, Silverglade began devoting his efforts to Gleason's full time. In 1987, he started running live boxing cards at Gleason's Arena, which was located one block away from the gym. That lasted until 1990, but Silverglade remained involved in the business side of boxing as a matchmaker and booking agent.

He helped to promote the first world title fight in Russia as IBF Cruiserweight Champion Al Cole defended his title against Glen McCrory. He has also made fights for some of the game's top attractions: Arturo Gatti, Regilio Tuur, Vinny Pazienza, Mark Breland, and Zab Judah.

Silverglade is married and has two boys. He lives in New York City. He graduated from Gettysburg College in 1968 with a degree in economics. He holds a master's degree in the Sweet Science.